Love
Britten Ormiston

Unspoken Truths About Life After Birth

A Book About Post Pregnancy, Tips for Survival, Marriage and More!

*The Day to Day Living That
No One Prepared You For...
Until Now!!*

Britton Ormiston

Bloomington, IN authorHOUSE® Milton Keynes, UK

AuthorHouse™
1663 Liberty Drive, Suite 200
Bloomington, IN 47403
www.authorhouse.com
Phone: 1-800-839-8640

AuthorHouse™ UK Ltd.
500 Avebury Boulevard
Central Milton Keynes, MK9 2BE
www.authorhouse.co.uk
Phone: 08001974150

This book is about personal experiences of childbirth, daily living and marriage. I am not a practicing medical physician and I do not suggest practicing 'home remedies' without your doctor's advice. <u>*Always*</u> *seek the advice of a physician for any concerns or ideas when treating yourself or your children for ailments.*

© 2007 Britton Ormiston. All rights reserved.

No part of this book may be reproduced, stored in a retrieval system, or transmitted by any means without the written permission of the author.

First published by AuthorHouse 1/17/2007

ISBN: 978-1-4140-5734-7 (e)
ISBN: 978-1-4140-5733-0 (sc)

Library of Congress Control Number: 2006906779

Printed in the United States of America
Bloomington, Indiana

This book is printed on acid-free paper.

On The Cover: *Sonogram picture on front cover was taken by Dr. Thomas Goggin, Athens, Georgia. 2002/2003*

This book is dedicated to my beautiful children:

*Julia: "The Grasshopper"
and
Nathaniel: "Nater the Tater"
and
Justin: "Bit-Bit"*

Acknowledgements:

I could not have written this book without the support of my family and close friends. I would like to thank my sister and my mother, both of whom are constant fixtures in my life. They put up with my quirks and specific requests and still love me. I also owe thanks to many of my friends who have shared their personal experiences about their lives and children. I would like to recognize my colleagues who tolerate and appreciate me for the person I really am.

Thanks to my loving mother, brother, and ex-husband who LABORED through editing every feminine topic of this book and survived! Also, thanks to my Dad who supports my every dream.

Lastly, I would like to thank my husband, Marc, and children. I could not enjoy the roll of motherhood and life so completely without them!

TABLE OF CONTENTS

Preface
1

Chapter 1
"In the Beginning…"
5

Chapter 2
"Aliens in the Mist"
9

Chapter 3
Demand It, It's Your Life!
13

Chapter 4
What REALLY Happens Once You're at Home
27

Chapter 5
The Feminine Stuff - Must we really?
41

Chapter 6
The Dreaded "Back to Work"
49

Chapter 7
Breastfeeding and Pumping
67

Chapter 8
Best Buys, Good Ideas and Pass em' On!
91

Chapter 9
When They're Sick!
107

Chapter 10
Don't forget about YOU!
117

Chapter 11
Can this Marriage Survive?
121

Chapter 12
You can Make it!
155

Epilogue
159

PREFACE

There are several reasons for writing this book. My main objective is to be able to reach parents and share with them the advice and helpful tips I have learned along the way from my family, friends and physicians. I really want to tell each of you not to be afraid of what is happening as you progress in parenthood. You must be sure to reach out to the network of people around you for help and support.

I am amazed at the number of working mothers who have moved away from home and left their network of life-long friends behind. These mothers venture out in the world in hopes of starting a new family. When their first child is born, they do not have anyone to tell them the specifics of what to expect in their NEW life.

These are REAL-LIFE stories of what you might expect to happen after having your firstborn, including situations such as needing answers to questions at two o'clock in the morning when there is no one to call for help. I hope to reach out to mothers who do not have anyone to give them the 'skinny' on how things really happen in life.

Another objective for writing this book is to tell you about bargains and 'must haves' for your family. We have all spent countless hours searching for the perfect items for our children. What's the safest? What did your girlfriend buy? Why? Was it reasonably priced?

I will give reasons for why I purchased a particular item, how I found it, and what I like about that item. Hopefully my reasons will help take the 'guess-work' out of your quest in buying the perfect items for your child. Some examples of perfect items discussed are bed rails, children's books, toys and vehicle accessories for children.

Be sure to check out my "<u>Note to Reader</u>" and "<u>Good Tip</u>" sections in this book for helpful information on many topics.

I want to give you "motherly" advice about breastfeeding, baby acne, diaper rash and other related topics. I don't know every detail. However, I have paid doctors, called my sister in the middle of the night, and struggled through different ailments with my children. All this time I've wondered 'WHY HASN'T SOMEONE TOLD ME THIS <u>SIMPLE</u> <u>STUFF</u> BEFORE NOW!?'

I hope to help working parents feel less stressed about the "have to's" of each day so that you can start enjoying the <u>little</u> time you have with your children. I will share my views on daycare centers. I want to tell you how to survive them if you must have your children attend a daycare center. I also will suggest alternative child-care options and "mommy child-care" strategies that could be quite beneficial for you emotionally and economically if you plan to work thirty to thirty-five hours a week on your job.

I want to tell you how much it means to hear other parents speak out about the same trials and tribulations that my family has gone through. Unfortunately, most families experience situations of isolation and shame and never seek help from friends or others (counselors, ministers, mentors, etc.). On a personal note, I can tell you that a similar pattern of non-communication is found in every marriage and the pattern is not dependent on social status or economic wealth. Marriage IS NOT an easy process without children. When little ones are added to the mix, the process becomes more compromising and difficult. I hope this book will provide an informational reference to console you and let you know you are not alone in your venture for the perfect family.

So on that note……..let's get started……..

CHAPTER 1
"In the Beginning…"

I live in a college town where many parents work and live in a University setting. I love it here! The air is clean, the campus is absolutely beautiful and the restaurants here are heavenly!

Many people in the Athens area are transient. I moved to Athens in the summer of 1990 to attend college at The University of Georgia. I had no idea I would still be here ten years after college. My intent was to graduate, go home, get married and live "happily ever after." -Funny how life didn't quite turn out like I envisioned.

Much to my surprise, I found a new and enjoyable life for myself here. Yet, every day life does have ups and downs. As a 33 year old, I feel I have experienced so many things in my life already. The older I become the luckier I feel to have transitioned into successful adulthood without losing everything, including the shirt on my back. Life is what we make of it. Sometimes breaking out of the mold of other's expectations and getting on with your life is the only way to make your life your own!

Now, I am a mother of three biological children working for the United States government. I put in forty hours a week at work and try to juggle both motherhood and work-life while keeping a smile on my face. Frankly, most days I want to scream. Some days I do scream!

Usually, though, I work at it until I find a balance between my 'two lives.' Then when my head hits the pillow at night I look back on the day and say "well done."

So, how do I do all this?
WITH A LOT OF HELP!

I don't know when Americans changed from a society where mothers stayed at home and raised children to a society of families who care more about what they bring home in their wallets than the quality of their home life. We are all passing our days being crammed in an office, a lab or a car for the sake of making a few extra dollars! We all do it day-in and day-out because our society demands it. Realistically speaking, in today's world, two incomes are necessary for most families to have nice things. -So, how then do we make decisions now that permanently shape our days of tomorrow? Very carefully!

Our Children's Innocence:

We should all realize that innocence in a young life lasts for a fragile moment, only a 'drop in the bucket' of time in what we parents experience with our children. Someday, we will look back at our teenagers and wish we could start over as parents, but with knowledge and experience! We should enjoy <u>EVERY MINUTE</u> we have with our children, especially in their younger years, for we cannot ask for that time back.

When I was pregnant with my son and still carrying my young daughter in my arms, I was approached by three older women on separate occasions. All three women had the same message. Their message was: ***"Raising your children will be the best days of your life so enjoy them now and don't take them for granted!"*** *Their message stays in the back of my mind as I worry about how I will raise my children. I wade through my days hoping for a way to find freedom and fortune in this life as a "working mom." Everyday I wake up and I feel I **am not** enjoying anything other than my children's smiles and an occasional decent night's sleep. I hear a desperate voice inside me say, "I want to change my life! I want to live again!"*

Changing our lives is always a work in progress, never beginning or ending. Finding balance in one's life is possible. However, you have to be willing to do things you said you would never do. You have to be willing to try things you said you would never try. You have to accept that a lot of the things your parents told you are actually true. You have to be willing to give a lot of yourself and ask for help when you need it! Last, realizing and accepting that when things seem perfect, life will inevitably change in an instant and place you back at 'square one.'

Once you can respond to life's changes with an open mind and flexible schedule, then you have truly started working your way toward the 'perfect parent.'

I haven't mentioned children yet. The reason why is simple: your children are only one of the factors in your new life called "family." However, they will become a parent's single most important focus from the moment they are born until the time they leave the household (and even long after that....).

My mother has annoyed me in years past with her sappy and sentimental stories of how she raised my siblings and me. She said I wouldn't understand the complications of parenting until I too became a parent. At my young age, I felt I knew as much as she did. How dare she think she was more knowledgeable than me or that she existed at a level of maturity that I couldn't understand?

***Well, okay mom, the cat is out of the bag.....YOU WERE RIGHT!

CHAPTER 2
"Aliens in the Mist"

Recently, my sister (Molly) and I were chatting about our lives over the phone. I said to her, "You know Molly, so many women are struggling through life trying to figure out how to care for their children and have absolutely no clue what is going on!" Her response was, "As a parent, why does everyone look at me like I'm an Alien? -Or some foreign person who is talking gibberish when words come out of my mouth? I want what's best for my kids and I am only a mom trying to relate these simple wishes to others. People simply just don't understand me until they too experience parenthood for themselves. Life after having a baby is such a different world."

Why did she make the above bold comment about people without children?

I used to think my sister was an exaggerating "know it all" who went on and on about bargains, runny noses and medicine for her kids. No doubt, I respected her and admired her greatly, but I was stuck in my "no parent" life- style and couldn't relate. Please don't think that I didn't enjoy my nieces and nephews. Rather, I was just separated from their daily rituals and routines. I had no way of knowing the pressures a mother faces every day. I didn't have that natural instinct which tells one to tuck their child under their wing to protect them from everything no matter what. I couldn't imagine getting up off the couch from my nap to go change a dirty diaper, fix a bottle, or give someone a bath. Watching Molly cut her children's food into bite size miniature morsels for her "baby birds" to eat was annoying. Give me a break!

Until....

"Until you have your own, you simply just don't know."

Okay, so this is not to insult or belittle those of you who have a wealth of baby knowledge and a true abundance of love for children despite the fact that you are not a parent. However, one is merely an outsider (no matter how much we like to think we aren't) until you create that bond with that special little someone new who captivates your heart and turns your life inside out. I am talking about the creation and pure joy of having a newborn child and also the way they change everything inside your heart. I'm not talking about the physical changes in your living arrangements or how difficult things can be when you have a newborn enter into your daily routines.

I was always angered when someone would say, "Oh, you better get as much sleep as you can because you'll never sleep again once you have that new baby," or, "Your life will never be the same once the baby is born."

Okay, these comments may be true but enough already! I always said the best piece of advice I could ever give a soon to be first-time mom was **"take everyone else's advice, mine included, with a grain of salt."** We are all different individuals and things that worked for you and me may not work for another new parent."

<u>Bottom line:</u> You must figure out what things work for you! Make those things a part of your daily life to regain control, composure, and put a smile on your face.

I am going to get on my 'soap box' and gripe about American life again (I will do this periodically through out the book, so bear with me).

Who is in charge of the curriculum needed to teach our children basic morals, values and everyday living knowledge?

Too bad we don't have courses in school available on social relationships, money management, married life and life as a parent. Aren't these truly the things we most encounter in our daily lives? English, math, history and science are important to our children's growth towards their professional future. However, we are lacking the specific education to help our children learn how to deal with the ups and downs of family life. Though it should be the responsibility of the parent[s], today's parent doesn't have enough time to spend teaching these basic morals and values to our children. No wonder there is so much divorce and separation from friends and family in the world today. We aren't taught how to get along with each other anymore. Family simply becomes only our husband and children.

What family? Yes, you have brothers and sisters with children. Remember your nieces and nephews? You have grandparents, parents, and even an aunt or uncle thrown in the mix. And remember those cousins we rarely see and don't socialize with because we are too busy to take the time to connect?

I am saddened by our lack of commitment to our extended family, to our loved ones, to our parents and to each other. We all need to focus as human beings on what I believe is the true nature of why we are on this planet. -To enjoy and love your whole family FIRST, then your friends and everything else should come after that. Material wealth should only be a distant third to your enjoyment list. Quite honestly, financial wealth usually accompanies your harmonious life only after you have all other areas in place.

In my opinion, in order to get back to what really matters in life, we should start at the beginning of one's "new life." This life consists of a pregnant woman who is somewhat lethargic, very tired of visiting the bathroom twenty times a day and being bloated, and two days away from bursting at the seams if she doesn't get her infant out of her womb…..

Let's get to business!

CHAPTER 3
Demand It, It's Your Life!

I have to give my sister credit for being my savior because when it comes to motherly advice she has always been able to answer my questions. My sister is a natural born doula (a personal caretaker for mother and child during labor and after the birthing process). I honestly feel I could not have made it through the birth of my children without her.

I shudder to think of the mothers who do not have a seasoned individual with them during the birthing process. I know, I know! I also felt it was too private a moment for the "common wealth" to view my private areas while waiting for the birth of my child.

However, things change!

*I told my sister half-way through my first pregnancy that I only wanted Kurk to be in the room with me when my first child was born. After all, my body is a private matter, and I didn't want the world seeing it! Yes, she is the "world" in my eyes! So is the doctor but he **had** to be there. Molly never pressured me to be present during the birth of my child. However, toward the end of my pregnancy I was afraid of not having a person in the room that had gone through the birthing experience (besides the doctor of course). What if Kurk passed out or I needed her to help me push?*

My sister is a mother of two children and has been <u>actively</u> present for more than sixteen births. Molly's experience of helping mothers go through the birthing process seems to come to her naturally. I discounted my sister's valuable experience until I was faced with giving birth to my own child.

Finally, I asked Molly if she would accompany Kurk and me in the delivery room for the birth of our first child. She happily agreed. Fortunately, one of her strong points is she is never pushy. She lets me decide what is best. She does make subtle suggestions but never crams them down my throat.

So we're off....the day of labor induction...

At 5 A.M. we arrived to register at the hospital. The hospital should have had my information already with my pre-registration/admission form, right? Wrong! They didn't have a single piece of information on me. It took the greater part of an hour to register and get up to my room. To make a small note about the early morning, I had already given myself an enema. Lord forbid my bowels would release while giving birth to my child while everyone in America was watching (that's how I felt!). I had gas and an upset stomach because the enema was of course doing its job. Molly and I were rolling in laughter because it really was a comical scene. We made it to the room after registration and I received an I.V. and a heart beat monitor for the baby. I made trips back and forth to the bathroom because I couldn't stop the diarrhea and gas. I was certainly worried about losing my continence on the table thanks to the diarrhea. About 6:15 A.M. the doctor came to administer the pitocin®. Pitocin® is a drug used to induce labor. It worked like a charm for me. About 8 A.M. I started having small labor pains......

Around 12 P.M. I'm in pain! "Where is my epidural? Help!" I could not believe that I was going through this pain and no one was doing anything about it! I had made it very clear to the nurse before receiving the pitocin® that I wanted every drug possible at every interval. "How in fact could it be then that I am still feeling pain?" "Drugs only assist in easing the pain, they don't make it a cakewalk," I was assured by one nurse. I finally get my epidural. I felt instant relief! I mean to tell you, my hat is off to those who wish to have the baby naturally (Are you crazy?). I am a strong willed, fairly tolerant to pain type individual, but this was down right scary! After my epidural was administered, I did great. My mom, my sister, my husband and my doctor sat around waiting for the big moment. It took a total of 10 hours to deliver my firstborn daughter, Julia. Dr. Goggin, Kurk and Mom were hot and heavy into a crossword puzzle when the time came for me to push. When it was time to push, we nearly had to pry the men away from one puzzle clue that was driving them nuts.

Pushing was difficult! I took all the classes, read all the

> **NOTE TO READER:**
>
> It never occurred to me that the delivery room would have a very earthy smell (Duh! Blood and the birthing process is an earthy procedure). I recall the smell of the room being not noticed or spoken of when I entered the birthing room during Molly's labor with her son. I didn't notice it when I was giving birth to my children but of course I was the one producing the smell, so go figure.

> **BIG FAT FLAG:**
>
> Why don't the doctors say something to you, why don't the nurses say the right things to you? Instead they all say, "....push down to your bottom...." Who talks like that? I know they are trying to be polite, but that means nothing to me.

books (I mean all the books) and did the Kegels. Even so, nothing prepares you for the real meaning of **P-U-S-H-I-N-G**. Okay, most nurses say, "Push down to your toes, curl up in a 'C' and count to ten and then take a breath and count to ten again." What the heck is that? I practiced and really tried to envision pushing, yet when the time came to push, I was in trouble. I couldn't seem to get the pushing down (pardon the pun here).

After about 45 minutes with no success, Molly asked for a mirror.

I asked her recently why she didn't jump in sooner to help me.

She said she was afraid of taking away from the experience that we were having. She didn't want to seem bossy or a "know-it-all" by telling me what to do. – So, she stood back.

Finally, the nursed asked Molly to take her spot while she left the room, and things got rolling. We got the mirror and placed it at the foot of the bed. Kurk and Molly each held one of my legs. Molly said, "Okay, I want you to lean forward and take a deep breath. Now, push down in the lower part of your stomach like you are taking a really big dump you are trying to get out, but can't (she pushed on my stomach to indicate the area right below my overstretched belly button)." I pushed correctly after her instruction and Julia was born within forty-five minutes.

I was frustrated and tired. Molly came to my aid. I needed her and she was there. Thank God someone could help, because I was helpless!!!!

After Julia was born, I can remember one thing……

-everyone disappeared. I had just been sewn up from tearing a tad. I was devouring a Chick-fil-A sandwich while still on the delivery table. I suddenly looked up and noticed I was alone. What a strange feeling! For an indefinite amount of time which seemed like forever, I was alone. Julia was gone, Kurk was gone, Mom and Molly and the doctors and nurses......-all gone. I didn't like feeling so alone, but how could I move? I was still numb from the epidural, so I sat there. Kurk was busy with Julia's first bath. Finally, Molly returned after only a few minutes.

Molly started helping me right away. She got a nurse who said I would be moved to my own room in a few minutes. Once comfy in my room, I found out the nurses had already ordered me a meal from the hospital...... -Good ole' french fries and a classic hamburger. When they delivered the food via room service, I devoured it without a second thought. I was very hungry! I rested while Molly situated my belongings. She began asking the nurse where things were in the building like the ice-maker, break room, nurses' station and any thing else on our floor that might be needed.

Why was it her business to ask all these questions?

Well, I'll tell you why: Molly was the only one who truly cared about my comfort for the next 24 hours. Thank goodness for her knowledge and persistence to get ice wrapped in a glove every few hours to control my swelling.

NOTE:
Using an ice pack for the first 24 hours can greatly reduce swelling.

Although the nurses do check your vital signs on a regular basis, they do not have a plan to make you personally comfortable. You have to express your physical needs out loud or suffer through the pain in silence. Make your own timed intervals where you ask for medicine, ice for swelling, and assistance in going to the bathroom.

> **NOTE TO READER:**
>
> I can remember when Molly's best friend had her first baby. When I walked in to the room after delivery, she was shivering from head to toe. I was told that placing ice "down there" caused the shivering but helped to ease the pain and swelling. I thought, "How odd! That's got to be cold and uncomfortable!" -Well, believe me, it is not cold! It feels great and is a necessity to keep the swelling at a minimum. The tissues around the birthing area are so numb from child birth that the ice is applied to relieve swelling (and not necessarily pain) at that early a juncture after birth. Most doctors say you will have a little swelling "down there." I tell you, my crotch felt like the size of a golf ball! It even inhibited my stride while walking which explains why most women walk so darn slow after delivery. The swelling is located right in between where your anus and your vaginal canal join. This area is commonly referred to as the "taint" and possibly may be subject to hemorrhoid pressure due to pushing.
>
> Many of my friends who have not experienced the birthing process were unaware that swelling of the vaginal tissues occurs after giving birth. Nor did they realize that ice packs were actually placed on the inflamed tissue for swelling after childbirth. Why not? I didn't know either! Why aren't we being educated on these topics?
>
> -And one more thing….Molly's friend wasn't shivering due to the ice. She was shivering because her body was releasing mega doses of hormones post delivery. People's bodies react differently to the stresses of giving birth: some people throw up, some people get nauseous, some people shiver, and some people are just fine…

How did I feel after giving birth?

I'm in the bed and just when I started to relax and rest......-"Um......"

I said "Molly, I'm not feeling so well!" In an effort to increase my comfort, Molly raised my bed with those wonderful mechanical lifting buttons. Unbeknownst to her, the raising of my bed was the last straw. I ran to the bathroom (as fast as a swollen post-pregnant woman could run) and heaved my guts out! The nurse walked in and said, "Well, honey, what happened to you? You were doing fine until now!" I felt like saying, "What do you think happened to me? I ate two meals because I was ravenous and hadn't eaten in 24 hours. My stomach could not handle all of the grease because of the post delivery hormones and I puked my guts out, what's it look like?"

In the bathroom I realized not only was I throwing up, I was bleeding from my posterior. Okay, I had been told about the bleeding in a somewhat nonchalant manner: "Just some bleeding for the next ten days. Then the bleeding should go away gradually until it turns brown to pink." <u>Sure!</u>

I was astounded to discover lots of my friends did not know that you bleed after you have a baby. The bleeding may

> **NOTE TO READER:**
>
> Don't do what I did. Don't eat a meal that is heavy with grease right after giving birth. I ate two greasy meals to add insult to injury. I would follow with a light meal that is easy on the stomach instead of a heavy meal! Not to say any of us pay attention to the "Have crackers and soup or a light sandwich..." statement when we are preparing for birth. In this case it will pay to follow my advice after delivery (especially if you have already thrown up during delivery) and start slow with foods easy to digest.

last up to three weeks as was the case in my personal experience. I made the mistake of packing my suitcase full of pretty nightgowns, magazines and things to do in my spare time. Why do the books tell us to do that? I ended up bleeding all over my nightgowns and didn't read one magazine! -Nor did I have time to do anything other than lay there and recover, try and learn to breastfeed Julia and greet the many, many visitors that had come to see my firstborn.

On a more personal note, no one bothers to tell you the 'standard' procedure for going to the bathroom after having a baby:

Go into the bathroom and hang your hospital gown on the back of the door to keep it out of the grizzly blood path. Now, take your little peri-squeeze bottle (*looks sort of like a bottle used to squeeze hair permanent solution onto the head, having a pointed tip for application*) filled with warm water and GENTLY squirt the water on your crotch area to loosen bloody debris. Dab your swollen skin with a dry, soft washcloth. Don't worry about the blood on the floor and everywhere else it is dripping, this is normal for everyone (you may even pass golf ball sized blood clots). Once you've dabbed to a semi-dried point, take the gigantic pads provided and place the pad on your net underwear. THANK YOU hospital industry for these fashionable drawers, they are great! Next, put two witch- hazel cleansing pads down the center of the sanitary pad. Place a medium sized glob of hemorrhoid cream or foam down the center of those two witch-hazel pads. Last, place your hand underneath your net underwear and pull up each side of your underpants to get them on your body. If everything you just placed on the pad doesn't fall off then you are ahead of the game! The pad itself may drop off with everything on it, so ask for help if you aren't modest. Pulling your underwear up for the first day is quite an accomplishment in its own right! If you've gotten this far, you're already doing better than I did. Put your hospital gown back on and make it to the bed. -Mission accomplished!

Once back in bed, try to rest. Do plan on having someone sleep in the room with you if you intend to keep your baby in your suite. You would not want to fall asleep and leave your little one unattended in the hospital. If you choose, you can send your newborn to the nursery while you sleep. The nursery is designed to take care of your newborn while you rest.

> **A WORD OF CAUTION:**
>
> Be SURE the nurses understand your wishes to breastfeed or bottle feed your newborn. One of my friends specifically told the nurses that her baby was only to be breastfed. Later that evening, her baby was given a bottle of formula while in the nursery because he "appeared to be hungry." Yes folks, this happened in a reputable hospital. So, make sure someone you trust is looking out for your little one and that your wishes are being fulfilled while your child is taken care of in the nursery.

You should be nice, positive and friendly when asking questions to the nurses. The hospital staff is not there for you to stomp on. The nurses help keep the hospital running and without them doctors would have a hard time serving as many patients as they treat daily. Most nurses are very nice but they do not know your personality and therefore may not recognize when you are in need. The nurses may also push you to your limit as they try and help you progress toward going home in good health. This is their job! Being annoyed when a nurse demands you feed your baby at a certain time while she watches the baby latch on your nipple is just one example of a nurse helping you progress. How about when you feel like buzzing them for the tenth time in two hours to ask them to complete another medial task which you are unable to accomplish on your own? You definitely fear your call may get on their nerves, so instead you suffer in pain. This is when that extra person comes in handy. -The girlfriend, the 'Molly,' the doula like individual you can count on. Your top choice of your 'doula' may be your husband, your best friend, your sister, or your mother. Your 'doula' must possess the confidence to speak up about questionable service and the ability to tend to your needs while you are recovering from birth. Additionally, you should feel comfortable asking this person to wait on you 'hand and foot.' Words cannot express how important this person is to your mental and physical well being during this time. Your hospital stay during your child birthing experience may not be as enjoyable if you do not have the network of support that every new mother needs.

> **NOTE:**
> **GRAPEFRUIT >>**
> **TOMATO >> GUM BALL**
>
> Your cervix will be about the size of a grapefruit after giving birth. Frequent checks of your cervix are necessary to make sure the swelling is decreasing. Your cervix should shrink considerably by the time your hospital stay is over and will gradually descend back to its normal place, below the belly button. After a few months of post-pregnancy, your cervix will be about the size of a gum ball (2-4cm).

Always stay the full length of time that you can at the hospital. Why?

Once you get home, you do not get the kind of care and attentiveness that you would and do get in the hospital. Unless you make your mind up to just rest in bed, you end up getting up from bed and doing more than you should at home. Being in the hospital gives you a chance to rest and let your body begin to heal from the birthing process.

Be sure to ask for extra supplies before heading home from the hospital. I asked for extra net panties and rinsed out the ones I had used while in the hospital to take home and wash. Try to get extra sanitary napkins, bed liners, foam and witch hazel pads before leaving the hospital. The hospital staff may drag their feet so ask for these items at different times during your stay. A good nurse will usually try to fulfill your request as soon as you ask for the items. Rest assured, you are paying plenty of money for your hospital stay and getting a few extra supplies will not make a big difference. Having these extra items in hand will allow for one less stop on the way home for your newborn's first car ride.

My second pregnancy, I took very few items to the hospital. My camcorder, baby bag for the baby, and everything else, all fit into one bag. I did not see the need to make checking out such a huge event. With Julia, it took two loads from the room to get the car packed with all the flowers and extra gifts. After Nate's birth, my cargo was at a minimum so that I could leave the hospital much easier.

One thing I remember vividly from my second pregnancy that I had forgotten from the first pregnancy was the utter pain I felt in my back and shoulders after the birthing process. For the first week home from the hospital it was so uncomfortable to just lie in bed without tossing and turning. It takes about a week for your back to stop aching and the time in between can be miserable trying to get rest at night. This time around I used the ThermaCare HeatWraps® (by P & G Products) which can be purchased at local retail stores.

Priced reasonably, they were well worth the money because the heat was perfect and the soothing comfort lasted an extended period of time while I was in bed or moving around the house.

Also be sure to take your Tylenol® and Motrin® at the correct intervals. Although I am one to balk at taking medicine, I always feel better after I take it. The trick is to take the medicine continually at the same intervals so it can work through your system and keep your swelling, pain and nausea to a minimum (taking medicine with ibuprofen has a cumulative effect which builds on the previous dose, so make sure you time your doses to get the maximum relief).

The exhausting leave from the hospital makes you dream of your bed, but once home it isn't as carefree as you might think. First, you have to get home......

I can remember being so nervous driving home with Julia in the car for the first time. We had to stop by the pharmacy to pick up my prescriptions (which was not easy, have someone do this for you). By the time we got home we were exhausted from tacking on a few hours of the learning curve of first time parents getting the car seat in, not spilling flower water all over the car and just making it in the house with all the luggage.

It does feel great to climb in your own bed and relax, but this is when your NEW life has just begun......

FLOWER REMEDY:

Duh! Mom said to dump the water out for the ride and refill it when you get home, I would have NEVER thought of that, how simple!

CAR SEAT FIX:

The trick to putting a car seat in the car <u>correctly</u> is to place your knee in the empty car seat while the car seat is in the seat of your vehicle. Shift all your weight onto the knee which is placing pressure down on the car seat and push as hard as possible. Gather some extra seat belt slack BEFORE putting the belt through the back positions of the car seat and then take the seat belt and slide through the proper holes behind the sitting area of the car seat. Collect the extra slack from the belt once through the back of the car seat and then tighten the seat belt while still applying pressure to the car seat with your knee. At this point you should have to push with pressure to snap the seat belt closed, if you don't experience this pressure, you need to re-read and follow the steps above.

Once you remove your knee from the seat, check to make sure the seat does not have any movement. If the car seat does move, get a tether strap (which straps behind the adult seat to hold the car seat in place) or try a belt clip to hold the seatbelt in place so the seatbelt does not loosen after pressure is released. In general, belt clips are needed for older model cars (1990s).

CHAPTER 4
What REALLY Happens Once You're at Home

When I was growing up I envisioned this picture of having the camcorder pulled out, recording us walking up to the door and going in with the new baby, just like on TV. We were all smiling, all happy over our new bundle of joy and everything appeared dreamy. Once inside, I was whisked away to my resting quarters and waited on hand and foot. The baby was brought to me when I requested his presence for feeding time. My every need was taken care of and my family and husband got along like magic during their stay to help with the baby!................... ***DREAM ON!***

Though this picturesque scene really does come true for a few very lucky individuals, the rest of us are left with "Okay honey, we're home, you've popped that baby out, now let's get back to living!" These words may not physically be stated, but the actions surrounding the family members will prove them true. Next thing you know, you are cooking dinner all the while thinking you feel pretty good, "So it shouldn't be a problem." Then you're doing laundry and taking care of your newborn. The truth is: This is the first day of the rest of your life! Suddenly, you realize, *"Hey, I thought I was supposed to get the red carpet treatment here, didn't*

I just squeeze and eight pound watermelon out of a tiny orifice, does anyone care?????"

Most women choose to stay in the hospital now days, because once at home, they are treated as though their recovery is immediate and life can resume to "normal" living.

Thank goodness my mother was there for me after Nathaniel was born because I learned the hard way that women do need help after giving birth.

After having my first child I decided I did not need anyone to stay with me at home because Kurk would be there to help take care of my needs. When it came down to every task, I felt I couldn't ask for help because I feared he might think I was being too bossy and too lazy given my new motherly state. As a result, I suffered in silence a lot because I didn't want to inconvenience Kurk and get on his nerves. Honestly, that should have been the last of my concerns. I bet many other new mothers who haven't had help at home have experienced these same feelings.

> **BIG EYE OPENER FELLOWS:**
>
> Please know that not only is your wife mentally and physically exhausted, but her hormones are shifting all around and will for quite some time, making her full of energy one minute and flat out exhausted the next.

Where did my husband go?

I know many women are asking the same thing after giving birth to their children. Your husband does love you and does want to participate in your new life "with baby." The problem is that he doesn't know how he fits into the puzzle when your infant is so small. All the books say, "Give him the bottle and let him wake up and do the 2:00 A.M. feeding so you can rest." Yeah, right! I don't think many men feel that comfortable feeding their infant right off the 'starting line.' Nor do many men wake up in the middle of the night and feed a crying infant, much less even hear the baby crying. Taking care of a newborn is not something innate for most men. Husbands simply sleep and then reply later, *"Oh, yeah, I heard him crying last night…..,"* knowing wives will be the one to get up and take care of the newborn.

Suppose a parent, friend or sibling does come over to help you. This will leave the wife in a 'Catch 22.' If you do not get help outside the home you end up doing a lot of the work or taking care of your newborn by yourself. Asking for help for the simplest of tasks like keeping your water stocked and bringing you wipes for your infant's diaper changes are all part of the things you will need assistance with during the first few weeks at home. Suppose you do have someone over to help, your husband will then say, *"There was no room for me to help with anything. I was being ignored while everyone else waited on you hand and foot. Obviously, you didn't need me."* Next, we get the story of, *"Well, since I am not 'equipped' to feed the child I cannot be of any assistance to this baby until he/she gets bigger."* The old breastfeeding excuse is classic and one I bet is used often from fathers of newborns.

More honestly, I think the situation is that most men feel awkward about the whole "new baby" thing and how we as a family are going to deal with this change in our NEW living situation. Add in the complication of the fact that he is probably sex deprived because you haven't slept together in months due to your size and discomfort and you have a classic, "I feel left out" husband, and understandably so! So, being frustrated with one another in the first few days and weeks after childbirth, although very tiring, is another scene I see playing out again and again in families after childbirth.

After a few months the baby will grow and actually do something other than sleep, eat and poop. These are the moments the father will start to interact with their newborn.

Kurk must have thought Julia was like a fragile china doll because he wouldn't pick her up for months. He just looked at her and smiled, that was enough contact. It really began to irritate me and get on my nerves and make me feel like he just didn't love her or want to be around her.

Rather, I think men are not mentally drawn to a "meat loaf" (as one of my friends called their newborn) who did nothing but eat, poop and sleep all day. Women tend to be able to put up with a crying newborn with so many needs because it is a natural instinct, part of the reason we are the "mommy."

With my second child, Nathaniel, Kurk followed the same pattern, keeping distance while Nate was young. I was not as upset or offended about his reaction to Nathaniel because I knew in a few months, their relationship would change drastically. Some individuals have to find comfort within themselves and their ability to handle a newborn before they can comfort their child, as was the case with Kurk.

Bathing the slippery suckers: Are there any special instructions for bathing my infant?

I have a few tricks I would like to think make it a tad easier to bathe your child. First, be absolutely sure to have one of those 'bath cradles,' which looks like a slanted cot, to place your child on even as a tiny newborn to bathe him/her. I never bought a "baby tub" because it was a waste of money in my opinion. I did use the hospital pan to keep a reserve of water in the tub to dip the washcloth in. The water will not be deep enough in the tub due to your infant's small size, so the hospital pan full of warm water will suffice. Be sure to warm the base of the tub first and get the tub cradle warm. Place the infant on the cradle with the water running or already filled, doesn't matter. I put Nathaniel in a few times on a cold tub cradle and he would just about climb out of his skin in tears before I figured out that he wanted to be introduced to the water nicely, as we would treat ourselves.

I always start with the mouth. I wet the cloth with warm water and wipe the gums down first because I don't want to put dirty tub water in the baby's mouth. I think cleaning the gums is important because it helps keep the baby's mouth clean. Next, you need to be sure to clean the baby's body. Be sure not to get soap in his/her eyes. You can put your infant in the adult tub and carefully bathe them with out getting the umbilical cord area wet. Don't forget to wash their 'private parts.'

I see so many moms who are afraid to check and clean parts of their baby's body. Until your children learn how to do it for themselves, it is your job! Don't be afraid to clean the penis or the labia. Also, clean their hind end to make sure it is free of fecal matter. Rinse out the pee-pee area with water, and use a cloth to dab any foreign (cheesy) material out of his/her private area.

For little boys:

Nathaniel got this creamy, yellow, cheesy matter where he had been circumcised. I thought it looked like puss. However, the pediatrician said it was normal. I was very careful to <u>gently</u> dab his penis with a warm cloth and slowly loosen the cheesy matter from the skin. I did not mess with this debris too much at one time. During each bath, I was able to remove a little more each time. Be sure to never rub your child's privates with a wet cloth because it hurts.

Once you are finished bathing your child, always make sure that you have a towel readily available. Here are a few easy options on removing your child from the tub:

1) Set the towel on the edge of the tub and place the bottom of your infant on the towel in a sitting position, then wrap the towel around the infant.

2) Turn your infant in a cradled position with his face looking at the floor and place your hand around his stomach with the baby lying forward on your hand. Place a towel on his back, then turn him back over with the towel underneath him and wrap it around the front.

Baby rash:

Don't forget to dry every crevice and crack on your baby's body. Baby rashes lurk in little wet areas, so drying in between all of the baby fat rolls will really help eliminate moisture rashes.

> **NOTE:**
>
> The pediatrician showed me how to push back on the skin surrounding the penis head as the skin tends to attach and stick to the penis head after circumcision. I would push the skin back by placing a finger on each side of the penis and pulling the head of the penis gently outward (with my other hand) against the pressure exerted by my fingers. I did this once a day or as needed when I changed Nate's diapers in order to keep the skin of the penis from attaching to the head of the penis early after circumcision. If your child's penis hasn't had this technique done regularly, the initial "breaking" of the skin will leave a red raw looking ring right underneath the head of the penis if it is stuck to the skin. However, the pediatrician will break the skin sticking to the penis if you don't and the longer you prolong the fix, the more it will hurt later. Be sure to keep the skin pulled back daily. I found it took about 9 months for the penis to completely heal and stop sticking to itself after circumcision.

Here I have to tell you about two wonderful products: First, I am an avid user of Desitin® (by Pfizer)! I love the stuff. Did you know adults can use it too? It is such a wonderful cream. I can't say enough about it. I usually put Desitin® on my children's rump at night, even when they don't have a rash. Most parents wait until the rash is bad and they have to use an ointment. I may tend to over use it. However, I think of it as a thin layer of medicine protecting my children's skin from the pee-pee monster. You can even use it on the spots where the diaper may rub and create a red spot on the leg, or any other areas that seem to look rashy and painful. I choose to use the regular Desitin®. The Desitin® with aloe-vera doesn't seem to work as well for diaper rash on my children. Don't forget, when your baby boy has just been circumcised you need to squirt Vaseline® (by Unilever) on his penis in a big tall circle (much like when you get ice cream from a machine and place it on a cone). Dab the Vaseline® on if it starts to fall off the end of his penis. Your local retail store should sell Vaseline in little squeeze tubes instead of those square hard-to-use containers. Buy about 4 tubes of Vaseline®. That, plus the hospital supply will be plenty. Be sure to ask for extra supplies (remember?). I also liked to use the round cotton pads (commonly used for removing nail polish) to place over the Vaseline®/appendage site in an effort to keep his penis from sticking to the dry diaper.

The mushy mess:

Kurk came into the bedroom one day as I was changing Julia's diaper when she was an infant and said, "Hey, what's this brown stuff streaking down the closet door here?" I calmly answered, "Oh, that would be sh*t," and kept right on going with my chores. I was amazed because I hadn't even noticed the poop streaking down the white closet door!

Babies just tend to send that stuff flying and you just have to try your best to stay out of their target path. I have changed diapers many times in the first few months of my children's lives and gotten "blown out" by Julia or Nathaniel. For those of you who haven't experienced parenthood, the poop that you deal with in the beginning is more liquid (for breastfed babies) than solid. You have to be an artist to quickly switch from one diaper to another without getting a "blast." The feeling of fresh air on their little butt cheeks must send a signal to the brain letting them know it's time to clean out the 'ole' pipes'. Usually you'll try anything to stop this flatulence from hitting anything other than its intended target (the diaper). Hands go flying up, blankets get thrown over the baby, and an all out war is unleashed to stop the poop from getting all over the baby and you!

> **MEMORY**
>
> I had a girlfriend call me once, she couldn't figure out why her baby was sweating up his back at night (to the point that she would have to change him during the night several times). She was terribly concerned that he was sick, the house was too hot, or she just had a hot-natured baby. I was baffled because I didn't have experience with boys at this point, so I had no answers. - Off to "Doctor Molly." I picked up the phone and called her to ask 'what was up' with this situation. Molly laughed, then said, "Tell her to point her son's penis toward the side or down in the diaper." *Oh, duh! I would have never figured that out... I guess men position "themselves" all the time down there, so we've got to do it for our babes until they can take care of it on their own.* I called my friend back to give her the good news; that her son was in fact well and on the road to comfortable and dry sleeping nights again!

The good news is after about 3 months, the explosive pooping stage will decrease considerably. The need for so many diapers will lessen. In fact, you may find that your baby is not pooping at all, when before he was a natural "cannon ball." I was mortified when Nathaniel stopped pooping six times a day at 3.5 months of age. Don't get me wrong, I was pleased not to have to change so many diapers. However, I was scared something was terribly wrong! Molly assured me that it happened with Julia (and with her two children as well) but I certainly don't remember this sudden decrease in the pooping business. I got so nervous about his functions I called his pediatrician. His doctor told me about baby suppositories (laxatives) for children. I didn't have a clue those existed! They work do mind you. Now that I have gotten used to Nathaniel only pooping every other day, I am not subjecting his extremities to any more laxatives unless necessary. After about 5.5-6 months, their bowels will start to regulate and you will see a more regular consistency of poop as well as a regular diapering pattern develop for your child.

The simple things we forget as our children grow!

On the topic of diapers, I see so many people putting diapers on kids that are **too small**! I tend to put diapers on my kids that are too big! I would rather them "swim" in a diaper than have diaper rash around the legs because a diaper is squeezing their little limbs. Parents, one hint that the diaper may be too small is that the baby will start oozing poop out the side or top of their diaper. Usually that means there isn't enough space between his rump and the diaper itself, so it shoots out the side (occasionally this will happen no matter what you try, it's the nature of the 'pooping beast'). Don't forget to take your finger and run it along the inside of the "elastic" around the "leg holes" of the diaper once a fresh diaper has been placed on your child. If the elastic around the leg is not all pulled out the poop can escape. You will need to make sure that the diaper is straight on the leg and pulled out in a uniform condition.

Burning bottoms:

How do you feel after you've gone to the bathroom with an upset stomach and you have that acidy liquid left on your derriere? Not good huh? Well, I am sure babies feel the same way. After a bad bowel movement, be sure to clean with a wipe and wipe the child's bottom area thoroughly and follow with Desitin®. Even if it means wasting a diaper or two if your baby poops a lot, it is not worth the discomfort to your child. Diaper rash has come to be an "expected norm" for children. I say 'Nay!' and please pass the Desitin®.

A very red rash may form in the presence of severe diarrhea and could escalate to a yeast infection. After the diarrhea subsides the rash should clear up within a day or two. If the skin continues to look chard or burned and blood red after ample time has past, consider having your child checked for a yeast infection. Also, a bumpy looking, red dot appearance can signify a yeast infection. Both female and male children can develop yeast infections because of the presence of prolonged moisture and contamination on the skin. Red bumps around the mouth where a child uses a pacifier could likely indicate a yeast infection as well. Using the ointment mixture on page 39 persistently around the mouth and boiling pacifiers will help rid your child of yeast infections on the skin around the mouth. (Thrush is a completely different type of yeast infection on the tongue of a child or adult. The tongue will appear white and fuzzy and it will be somewhat painful to eat or swallow. An oral prescription must be administered to take care of this type of yeast infection). Yeast infections are often seen particularly after your child has taken prolonged medication from having a cold or being sick.

Belly button goop:

I think some parents might be afraid to get down in that belly button after the umbilical cord has fallen off. The black "umbilical cord goop" left over inside the belly button will come out. To get the goop loose, take a cotton swab and carefully clean out their belly button. You do not have to get it all at once, little by little, if you work at it each bath time, the black goop will dislodge.

Baby Ears, Toes and Nose:

You should not clean down inside your infant's ear drum area. You can clean the outside of the ear where the wax is designed to come out. Be sure to dry behind the ears and the area around the ears. This keeps water from building up in their ears which can cause ear discomfort and pain. Also, be sure to dry in between their toes. *Do you like putting on socks while your toes are still wet?* Don't forget to clean their nose out with a cotton swab if needed, they can't blow their noses like you and me!

Bumps, flakes, and peeling:

What are all the extra skin blemishes, redness, bumps and flaky-peeling going on with my infant's sweet newborn skin?

Well, it's probably cradle cap, baby acne and other newborn blemishes. How do you get rid of it? A friend told me her doctor said you have to wait it out, that it is natural and that you cannot get rid of it. Nonsense! You can! My sister took her children to a dermatologist because they have very sensitive skin. They can only use Cetaphil® products (by Galderma Laboratories) and Aveeno® products (by Johnson & Johnson). The children's doctor gave her an ointment recipe for their skin problems and told her to mix the ointments together at a one to one ratio. Carefully put the mixture on the baby's body wherever there is a skin condition. Don't use just a small amount; be sure to put enough to cover the area thoroughly (as you would when you put lotion on your skin to nurture a dry area).

Here is the recipe:

> Even amounts of:
>
> **Hydrocortisone 1% cream**
> to
> **Clotrimazole 1% cream (antifungal cream)**
>
> ***Mix with spoon or your fingers and put in Tupperware to store long term. Use after bath time and for cradle cap, baby acne, and dry red skin folds. Apply Desitin® over this ointment mixture to add a double layer of protection and healing.

We use it for baby acne, bumps, dry skin on the backs of knees, red flaky cheeks in winter, severe diaper rash and yeast infections, and cradle cap (just rub it right in the hair, so your baby's got a "gelled" hair style, so what! He feels better!), and many more ailments. Take care not to get it in the eyes. Now your newborn can look beautiful for those one month and three month portraits without all the touching up of the pictures! Enjoy!

CHAPTER 5
The Feminine Stuff - Must we really?

I'm sitting in the doctor's office with my feet in stirrups, which is an uncomfortable position as we all know. I had to deal with the scary fact that I had two pap smears returning with Class II results. It was enough to make my skin crawl. "What does this mean? Do I have cancer?"

I take good care of myself. I get regular check-ups, and I try my best to avoid carcinogens in our earthly environment (e.g.: second hand cigarette smoke, the sun and blackened foods from the grill, etc.). What the heck is going on here?

The Pap ain't all that:

The truth is the older we get and the more medical advances that are made, the more we should realize getting our pap smear results back with abnormal cells is going to become more common. Why? First, the testing methods for "precancerous cells" are becoming more sensitive because researchers continue to find new markers for cancer causing agents. Precancerous cells mean there "could be a chance" that your body will harbor a form of cancer in the future. Very rarely should you get a Class III pap smear classification on your results, which could be a bit more serious.

We must also take into consideration the human error factor. It is not unlikely somehow that your sample may have been contaminated and a second pap is needed to verify the results of the first.

So what's going on here?

During pregnancy, your body is going through numerous changes, not only chemically, but also physically. The lining in your uterus, your gums in your mouth, the skin on your stomach, your breast tissue to name a few parts, are going through severe morphological changes. These changes can last until the end of the breastfeeding period. Not uncommonly as did happen to me, I had a Class II pap smear classification result due to breastfeeding Julia. We went through the biopsy tests to find that really, the lesions in my uterus were due to changes during breastfeeding. These lesions disappeared after I finished the breastfeeding period with Julia. My doctor and I agreed that I wouldn't jump to conclusions and wouldn't perform any tests after the birth of my second child unless I had a Class III pap smear classification.

WORD OF CAUTION:

Each person is different and some people have an "I need to know NOW" attitude regardless of the severity of the pap smear results (Class II or Class III). In that case, don't cause yourself to have sleepless nights! Go and get the second pap smear or the biopsy. For those of us who have been through it before, wait until three months after breastfeeding and have the pap smear completed again. However, if you have a Class III pap smear, be sure to follow your doctor's advice.

I encourage each of you to really look at your medical history as a reference to why you could be getting these abnormal cell growth patterns. Also, talk to your doctor if you have any concerns.

Thankfully, after Nate's birth, my pap smear was normal. I have a feeling that some unrelated urinary issues I had after Julia's birth most likely caused the 'questionable cells' to show up on my pap smear.

It is also not uncommon to get a urinary tract infection after giving birth, so watch for signs of discomfort, unusually strong smelling odors, or pain in the stomach or back. Seek your doctor's advice immediately if you are not feeling well.

The more I speak with my friends about these personal experiences, the more I realize and accept that women are having less "normal" results on pap smears (pregnant or non-pregnant individuals). I sincerely believe this is due to the advancement of science, in which case I say, bravo! That means cancer or pre-cancerous cells can be detected that much sooner. You must weigh in your mind what medical practices you wish to follow so you feel good about any ultimate decisions you make about your body after pregnancy.

Cholesterol tidbit:

I was shocked and amazed after getting my results back from a physician that my total cholesterol was a whopping 245mg/dl, post pregnancy (anything below 200mg/dl is optimal and considered normal)! I couldn't believe it, I felt like a walking commercial for one of those cholesterol drugs you see on television where I appear to be in good health, yet I may keel over at any minute because my heart is screaming for a break!

Did you know that when you breastfeed, your cholesterol will normally be higher?

It is true. The liver will produce more cholesterol in response to a heightened level of hormones while pregnant (and nursing).[1] My doctor recommended waiting to check my cholesterol level again three months after I finished breastfeeding. Meanwhile, I am working hard at the gym to shape up my body and fight off any stress I am placing on my cardiovascular system.

Hemorrhoids:

Having a hemorrhoid is kind of like having the flu: You may think you've had the flu before, but once you've REALLY had the flu, you will never forget the unmistakable warning signs. Same rule applies for a hemorrhoid.

> **FAMILY HISTORY CAUTION:**
>
> Always remember that family history does play a role in our body's chemistry and ability to metabolize cholesterol. Therefore, don't assume that if you have high cholesterol during pregnancy, that it may only be pregnancy related. Diet, and exercise (or lack of) can also play important roles in your health. Be certain to discuss any cholesterol levels above normal with your doctor.

Hemorrhoids are very painful and by definition are swollen tissues and veins of the anus that often itch and burn when aggravated.[2] Did you know that processed foods can aggravate hemorrhoids? Lunch meats, hot dogs, and many more preservatives in processed

---

1 Donovan, Debbi, *Higher cholesterol levels when breastfeeding?*, http://www.parentsplace.com/features/heart/qas/0,,239248_106143,00.html

2 The American Heritage® Dictionary of the English Language: Fourth Edition. 2000, http://www.bartleyby.com/61/72/H0147200.html

foods can leave you in a 'heap of trouble' the next day. Be careful to recall what you ate the day before you had a "flare up" and be sure to avoid those foods in the future.

Hemorrhoid creams should help to ease the itching and are necessary for comfort and ease during the day. However, a true hemorrhoid will bulge outside your rectum. It can be excruciating to sit on when combined with all the aforementioned symptoms. My mom swears by about 600-800 mg of Vitamin B6 daily to help with this problem. The one time I had a REAL flare up, I was desperate for relief. I did try the B6 late in the game, but mainly I used the pads with witch hazel and the hemorrhoid creams for comfort and ease of itching.

You are not a Super Man....Woman!

It goes with out saying, don't try and lift a dresser on your own anymore! Okay, so you could lift a dresser when you were 15 years of age, even 20 years of age. Now as our bodies' age, we forget that when we sneeze, the pee can trickle down our legs (thanks to the loss of bladder control with pregnancy). Likewise, when we lift, the hemorrhoid can 'pop out' too, so be careful. Instead, ask that cute hubby of yours for help when moving the baby furniture around the room for the 100th time.

Hair loss:

Have you been standing in the tub washing your hair, and notice more of your hair is in the bottom of the tub than on your head?

About three to four months after your pregnancy, your hair will start to thin out. You had to produce extra amounts of hormones to grow a person inside you, thus it makes sense that you would have extra hair follicles in the 'growing' phase during your pregnancy. Once your body adjusts back to its normal hormone levels (three to six months after pregnancy), the hair follicles will stop the extra growth and return to their normal growing patterns. Hence, your hair will begin to shed as the hair follicles let go of the extra hair. This is a normal process for most pregnant women. However, it can be very alarming when you get that first hair brush full of your gorgeous locks. Don't worry because your hair will stop shedding after about six to nine months, proving that you may not go bald after all!

> **NOTE TO READER:**
>
> If you feel that you are losing abnormal amounts of hair you may want to have your blood checked for thyroid problems or hormonal imbalances. Meanwhile, be sure to take a daily vitamin to up your nutrients and get plenty of rest.
>
> I've had several friends who have associated large amounts of hair loss with taking diet pills too soon after birthing a child. It may be wise to stop your quest for dieting until your body's hormones level out a bit more and you are able to replenish nutrients your system needs to hold on to your normal hair growth. I think 6-9 months after childbirth is probably a safer range of time to allow your hormones and nutrients levels to replenish before attempting dieting strategies.

Post-pregnancy periods:

About one to one and a half months after I stopped breastfeeding, my period returned. The problem is that I am having a period every two weeks and the flow is very heavy. Will my period ever be normal again?

After you stop breastfeeding and you have already returned to taking birth control (which is normal for most of us at this stage), you will find that it will take several months for your period to return to a normal cycle or pattern. I was told by my doctor that sometimes break through bleeding can occur while taking birth control after pregnancy. However, I have found that the break through bleeding is more of a "normal process," the body's natural way of "resetting its internal clock," and not necessarily related to taking birth control.

I had three 'rounds' of bleeding a week at a time with one week in between each menstruation. This continued for a six to eight week span until my period returned to some what of a normal pattern. This has happened with both of my pregnancies regardless of which birth control I was taking at the time. So, give your body time to adjust, be patient and things will level out in most individuals.

CHAPTER 6
The Dreaded "Back to Work"

The topic of going back to work after having started a family was a very touchy one at my house. Every family member will feel differently about whether or not the 'right' thing to do after having a baby is to go back to work. Some of my friends say that they have to go to work to escape the monotony of staying home all day. Others say that they really enjoy their work and need that time away from home to have their "own life." Still, more often than not, most of my friends are stuck in the predicament I find myself in: *"If ONLY I could afford to stay home, I'd be there this very minute."* I say these words at least once a week, and yet, here I am working fulltime every day away from home.

I think the issue of "back to work" that women face these days is very two-sided and hard to address. First, if you are like me, you went to college to gain an education in hopes of landing a good career to make money for

> **LISTEN UP:**
>
> Being a full time "at home" mother is a job all in itself and one that receives little merit from those in the regular work force. As Americans, I'm not quite sure why we disrespect our 'At Home Parents'. Your spouse or relative is doing the best thing for their children by staying at home with them as long as they can during their children's young lives.

your household. Now that you've had children, your job becomes less of a priority.

Your children now hold the "#1" hot seat in your list of "to-do's." To complicate things, you really like your job, but find it increasingly hard to concentrate while at work. Not only do you miss your children, but you also have 18,000 errands floating around in your head while trying to complete a task on the job. This is the very essence of why women are stuck between "a rock and a hard place," when it comes to our careers.

I had a husband who whole heartedly believed that the kids being home with their mother full-time was not always in the best interest of the children or the mother.

His reasons were:

1) Children don't have the opportunity to interact with other children their age while at home;

2) Mother can lack motivation and willingness to do anything outside the home;

3) Mother can develop an increasingly bad attitude by spending 8 hours (plus) a day home alone with a two year old toddler. Everyone needs a break.

These reasons may have some merit, but they are not enough to scare me away from staying home full-time with my children if given the opportunity.

To further complicate matters, my ex-husband was under the impression that in this day and age, both family members needed to be working outside the home in order to maintain a substantial income for the household because the spending patterns of a family typically do not change once the baby arrives.

Some spouses can have a sarcastic and lazy attitude toward a mother's wishes to become a full time working mother at home. I understand that our society in this day and age require both adult partners in a family to work, but who said either spouse has a right to get angry at the other if a family can afford to keep one parent at home. I think many individuals do not value the "stay at home" parent as they used too. Rather, I think it was more accepted as the norm back in our parents' time of raising their children. Although I think the mother still wasn't respected for her stay at home work position then either. Whether it's staying at home or going back to work, either option does not have to be the "End of the World."

> **NOTE TO READER:**
>
> Lots of families CAN AFFORD for one parent to stay at home with their children, but refuse to lessen their "debt load" to make it happen. Remember, you are choosing your destiny, and by spending more money than you make will assuredly guarantee you will not be able to be at home full time with your children.

I have personally felt that going back to work during some points in my life was the "End of the World." I felt helpless, leaving my children day-in, day-out.

Well, here are some of your options in the "going back to work" phase of your life that you should consider:

1) **You can work out of your home on a part time or full time basis while watching your children.** If you choose to take this avenue, try to hire some help from time to time, whether you hire and individual to clean your house, or a person to watch your kids while you are still in the home. Working by yourself with blocks of time can be so much more productive than an "hour here or an hour there." Wait until after normal working hours and hire a teenager who can come over in the late afternoon/evening and watch the kids while you work in your office on the other end of the house.

2) **If you choose to go back to work in the career of your choice or field, outside the home, find good daycare for your children.** ALWAYS research when it comes to daycare and check on your children in daycare often to be sure the business is fulfilling its contract as stated when you originally went to tour the facility.

3) **You can work part time and explore options for part time daycare while still accomplishing the career you choose and time away for yourself.** If you choose this option, I strongly recommend making sure that both you and your partner agree on what your "obligations" are on the "home-front" when it comes to the household. More often than not, since you have some "free" time, your spouse may expect more "work" from you at home than is feasible. Be sure to talk about every category of home life from cooking to cleaning. This way, there is no assumption

made by the full-time working spouse that just because you work part-time, doesn't mean you have the rest of the day to clean house and run errands (although admittedly you will spend some of your time doing these tasks).

4) **Stay at home and raise your children while living on one income.** This choice will no doubt require some frugal and well thought out planning on your part. It is a doable option and many websites are available to help you learn how to shave your expenses to afford this route if you so choose. You need to make sure your spouse is comfortable with a parent "staying at home" and be sure to set some guidelines of the working spouse's expectations. Many working spouses will get upset if they come home after a long day of work and feel like you have "accomplished nothing all day," even if that really isn't the case. You have to be sure your marriage is strong and both partners are in agreement as to what is and what is not to be completed by the time the other gets home. As fundamental as this may sound, it really is necessary in order to avoid conflicts in the long run.

5) **Work an opposite work-schedule from your spouse and switch off providing daycare for your children within your own home.** I know of several couples who have tried this option and if the relationship between the husband and wife is strong, it can prove to be a great family resolution. Though minimal time is spent together as husband and wife, one must remember this is only a temporary fix to 'daycare' in a long term family/marriage. Your children will benefit by staying at home daily with one parent or the other. This parent-to-child interaction will help develop a

deep bond and will encourage your children to trust in the stability of a schedule. You could also consider minimal daycare for up to ten to twelve hours a week in your home by a trusted friend to help the second shift spouse from working too late at night. If the second shift working parent trades off watching another mother's children (i.e. the trusted friend I just mentioned) for a few hours a week, you can avoid daycare cost for those ten-to-twelve hours a week. In this scenario you can pay less daycare and enjoy more time with your children while providing them with play partners a few times a week.

Let's research the first avenue, **staying at home with the children and working inside the home.** Admittedly, it is easy to get lazy and slack off if you stay at home all day. Adding to the workload, mothers are now trying to work out of the home and watch the children at the same time. This concept is something I have learned is a very difficult process. My sister tried working out of the home and she said she was working 'around the clock' with no breaks of leisure time. If she wasn't cleaning or trying to get the kids to take a nap, she was working "on the job" doing paperwork. Because it takes much longer to complete one single "working task" due to the constant attention that children require, she would end up working well into the night. It doesn't stop there either. Then there is dinner to cook, laundry to clean, children to bathe, and books to read all before preparing for the next day. This type of schedule can be exhausting to one person, and something I hear more and more mothers are doing in an effort to stay home with their children as well as earn an income instead of going back to the traditional work place.

I must admit I would be tempted to follow suit and work from my home if the avenue were to arise while raising my children. Somehow, I know I can beat the odds of this working mom thing, whether working in or out of the household. I just have to plan strategically, and surely good things will come my way. Listen, I am hoping against hope that every idea I have in my mind will somehow pan out and bring in the money needed to support my family. ***I do not seek these funds in an effort to gain material wealth; rather I seek this fortune to give myself the opportunity to relax in parenthood and to enjoy the best time of my life with my children!***

If you choose the option of **returning to the work field**, you are then faced with the harsh and undeniable truth of daycare. I have a HUGE soap box to climb on here because I think that daycare for the young and old alike is lacking tremendously in this country. There is only one state in the USA at the present time which comes even close to supporting our elderly in the way in which you would want your own mother or yourself to be treated as we approach old age. Likewise, daycare for the young (newborn-4 years) lacks the educated supervision much needed for our children as we raise the next generation.

Daycare has many good aspects as an institution. First, there are the undeniable benefits of child to child interaction and play that are tremendously advantageous in the growth and learning experiences of our children. Second, the educational planning involved in daycare is usually very well thought out and carefully planned by the lead program specialist for the daycare facilities. A well managed daycare is hard to find. If you find one, you should stick to it until your child can enter into Pre-Kindergarten (usually at the age 4 years).

Unfortunately, the individuals hired in daycare facilities usually lack the knowledge and experience needed to teach our children. Time and time again I have seen the "lack-luster" attitude of teachers as well as their lack of desire to be there. These negative actions greatly reduce the possibility of children getting a positive learning experience from daycare.

Isn't it comforting to know you are leaving your child with someone who really is only there for a paycheck?

And a small paycheck at that! In America, we do not pay any "daycare" worker well, whether it is to nurture and care for the old or the young in our families. Furthermore, we do not give the workers any technical training on how to sterilize toys or nursing equipment, clean up a runny nose or an unexpected bowel movement, or how to wash hands from one patient or child to the next to keep from spreading any sickness or contamination. Sure, in theory these health practices in daycares are SUPPOSED to be covered with each staff member and carried out on a daily basis. In reality, however, the fundamental steps that need to be followed to ensure a healthy daycare are brushed over or done at the minimum level required by the staff.

I have yet to encounter a daycare that actually made me feel as though my child was more important than the next, or encounter a staff member who was willing to make sure that they didn't spread a cold from a sick child to my child. I was lucky if the staff even spoke to me or related to me on any level about what might be in the best interest for my child.

As a parent, you cling tight to the hope that your child can be placed in a particular 'teacher's group' who is responsible and happy to have a full time job. You then pray that teacher can fulfill every aspect of daycare duties as you see fit, because in reality, they are the surrogate parent while you are away. Multiply your hopes placed on this one individual by about 17 other mothers (times two because fathers count too) and you have four staffed individuals in a room with 16 plus infants who can't keep anything straight. They are running to and fro to lunch, so "fill-in" workers come in and relieve the regular staff, which adds to the confusion. They are also changing diapers, cleaning spit up, and feeding babies with bottles that they can't remember to which baby the bottle belongs! Put all these things together and it makes for a situation that I have chosen for my children not to take part.

Julia was in public daycare for almost a whole year and it was an awful experience for me. I know some mothers who rave about public daycare from day one, but I feel maybe those mothers need to take a closer look at what kind of services their children are getting before they toot anyone's horn, including their own. I did not feel good about leaving my child in public daycare for many reasons, yet it was my only option at the time. I didn't have a choice but to return to work to help supplement the household income.

The first day I went to tour the daycare, I peered inside the window from my car. I watched infants being left in bouncy seats, cribs, rolling around on blankets, and sitting in little stationary play stations. Some workers were busy about changing diapers (I noticed some weren't wearing gloves, though I knew they were supposed to as they changed the diapers), while most workers sat and gossiped with one another until a baby needed a lap to sit in or a bottle to sip. If someone's child spit up, they simply wiped it up and kept on going, no cleaning of any sort done to that area where the child threw up for the next child to place there hand in the same spot. Runny noses, and coughing babies added to the mix (who really shouldn't be there), and pacifiers and bottles going into mouths of wrong babies was just enough to make me sick! The daycare Julia attended was a very reputable daycare and one of the few that I felt comfortable to choose from to keep my precious child.

When I would walk into the nursery and see babies in cribs with runny noses, coughs and crust dried on their face, I would think, "You've got to be kidding me!" Yet the children were allowed to be there because they didn't have a fever. Julia was sick almost every other week starting from 6 weeks of age when she began to attend daycare. I cannot count on two hands the amount of colds, coughs and fevers she was exposed to from daycare.

Doctors, nurses and daycare workers tell parents that when our children get sick it is "good for them because it helps to build their immunities." *Oh yeah, try telling that to my pocket book!* Better still, try telling that to an exhausted mother whose up from one to four o'clock in the morning with a child who can't breathe in a lying down

> **NOTE TO READER:**
>
> Some parents will bring their sick child to daycare having already given them a morning dose of Motrin or Tylenol. The medicine will hold their child's temperature down long enough giving the parent time to at least get a half day of work in before being called to come pick up their sick child who "suddenly" has a fever of 101°F degrees or higher!
>
> Simply stated, most parents don't realize that when a working parent has daycare as their only option to watch their sick child, they will do whatever it takes to bring home the paycheck so that they can keep the household running. This is a sad and infuriating pattern because it stands to reason that every other child in the room will possibly get the sickness due to that particular parent's lack of consideration!

position, so she has to hold them upright while they sleep (let's remember mom has to go to work in the morning too). These situations happen daily, yet, parents still drop their children off to these "germ factories" day-in and day-out, because it is the only option they have for their children.

After about a year of public daycare, I switched to **daycare in the home of a lady in my hometown.** *This daycare option was a much more enjoyable experience.* First, you had the total convenience of dropping your child off easily and quickly with a person you knew would be keeping your child all day. No hassles, no instructions to a different teacher everyday, just the same mom day-in and day-out who knows your child almost as well as you do. These "baby sitters" who choose to watch kids in their home usually aren't licensed. Rather, they are mothers who have chosen to quit their full time job to be with their kids and now supplement their incomes by watching your children too. The good thing is that you usually get great peace of mind that is worth a lot of money. Your children are rarely sick and when they are, the sitter is very understanding. The mother will usually do her best to help you with any overtime you need her to work. Also, the mother will usually accommodate you when you need to have your children dropped off or picked up for some event (doctor's office, appointment for school, after school programs, etc.).

The bad news about "in-home daycare" is even though you try to instruct the mother watching your children on your parenting preferences, you are reluctant to say anything negative for fear you might upset them, and vice versa. This can cause hostilities to build from time to time because the areas of parenting differences are not addressed immediately to "douse the fires." Preferential treatment of the mother's children over your children may cause duress. Some mothers who choose to watch kids at home will only work off of their schedules and feel like you "owe them something" since they are keeping your children outside of a daycare setting.

The not so rough points are that you must make both your schedule and the sitter's schedule the same for holidays and time off. So, be sure to work out whether or not your sitter will be paid during any vacation period (yours or hers), holidays or extra time off.

Having said all of that, I believe this experience was very pleasurable! **Getting someone you like and trust is the key.** *We liked the person who kept our children very much and felt comfortable with her parenting skills and the way she treated our daughter.*

Then, I got pregnant with our second child. We decided to negotiate with our same home "baby sitter" to keep both our children. We negotiated and reworked the financial numbers until both of us agreed on the payment. Things were looking good. Problem was, she was pregnant too. We were carrying our children at just about the same time of conception. This posed a problem. As our due dates got closer, I began to feel trapped. How in the world was I going to get two children up, over to another person's house, and get to work by eight o'clock in the morning?

IT IS NOT EASY to get one child up and ready for the day and out the door on time, but two children could be a nightmare! My next option was to ask my mother to come and live with us and take care of the kids. She hesitantly agreed and moved in a few months later.

Soon after mom arrived to live with us, Nathaniel was born. **I can truly say from experience that the option of a "live in" helper has its ups and downs.**

You cannot beat the convenience and pure care that an individual gives your child/children in your home, allowing you to leave as early as needed even if to sneak in a trip to gym while the kids are sleeping. However, if you work far away from home, you most assuredly won't see your children during your long work day. This is a concern to most new mothers who choose to breastfeed during the day or would like the convenience of being able to get to their infant quickly for a short visit during lunch breaks.

You lose a lot of your privacy when a person comes to live with you. Privacy doesn't seem to be a big issue for me, but my husband had a hard time feeling like his privacy wasn't invaded. To complicate things, he always felt like he had to compete with my live in "nanny" for my time because mom and I got along so well and talked all of the time. He must have felt like a "third wheel" or something because lots of times I heard him say that there was no room for "us" in our relationship because I spent my extra time with my mother and kids. Plus, most people don't relish the thought of living with their own parents, much less their in-laws, so I really appreciated that Kurk was willing to try this option of daycare, if only for a little while.

Clearly, the best working option to choose if you only need a small income is a **part time position.** *I have worked part time after the birth of my first child. I found there was a greater balance between home life and my work life. I was able to complete my work in the office daily by 1-2 P.M. Then, I was out of the office and on the road to being a mommy well within the 2:30 P.M. range. I found this situation so comfortable because I could run errands on the way home and then once home start dinner, pick up the house and do some laundry. Most all of the busy work was done before Kurk walked in the door. Julia and I also had some play time together. I actually felt like I accomplished more at work, because when I was at work, I* *had a smaller amount of time to be there, so I had to focus on getting the job at hand completed so I could "get out the door."*

> **NOTE TO READER:**
>
> I made an Excel spreadsheet which is a record of the day's happenings for the sitter to fill out. This way, I could have a report of what happened with my children while I was at work during the day. I think this is a good way to help the working mom stay connected to their children. Additionally, it also lets you know your child's eating patterns, pooping patterns, and any concerns the sitter may have or medications administered during the day. I suggest you make a sheet for your children so that you can feel comfortable too while away from your child. Be sure to include nap times, breakfast and lunches (Did they eat well, some, not at all?) dirty diapers and any special considerations. Also, include your phone numbers directly on the sheet so they will have your numbers close at hand should they need you immediately. Then, just print out the sheet and make lots of copies and the person can use one each day to keep you up to date with your child's daily routine.
>
> **I have included a generic daily activity sheet in the back of this book for you to print out and use at your convenience.**

Mommy daycare:

Mommy daycare is the concept of 4-5 mothers participating and taking turns caring for each other's kids at one parent's home or "base campsite," everyday of the week (one week day for each mother). Now, this sounds tough, but actually the hardest part is finding a parent willing to lend their house to a "daycare" type atmosphere. *I had two parents eagerly wishing to participate with me, but no one would offer their home. I lived about 30 minutes* *from where most of us worked, so it wasn't optimal to choose my home for the "base campsite."*

I worked the numbers very diligently and you can take annual leave as well as one day a month 'Leave Without Pay' and come out better long term financially than paying daycare for one child for a year. Yes, you will lose some pay, but the amount of pay you lose should typically be about $2,000 less a year than daycare costs for one child. For example, if you spend approximately 7,000.00 on daycare a year, you should only lose about $5,000.00 a year by using annual leave and 'Leave Without Pay,' and you get to spend time with your kids! That's a $2,000.00 savings!!!!

The idea works like this: You don't charge each other daycare cost and you don't charge for the person who agrees to lend their house as the base campsite. All mothers/fathers would have to agree and adhere to a strict drop off and pick up time and the house would have to be cleaned up after the end of each day. Having a playroom available in the house would be a wonderful spot to house this 'Mommy Daycare' facility. The mother who keeps "daycare" that day is responsible for a set meal (and the costs of feeding the children that day). This mother will feed the children the same meal every week on their scheduled day of daycare. If the mothers plan the menus together, then they (your children) can get a different meal everyday and remain healthy and happy.

This idea is especially encouraging for a mother with two children. The benefits are awesome because you don't have to pay daycare and you get to spend time with your kids while your children interact with other kids their age (and of your choice). *Every mom I talked to said it was a great idea, but because these waters were uncharted, I only had one other mom who was willing to "jump off the boat" and try it with me. She soon moved out of town and so this Mommy Daycare idea never came to pass.* However, this idea would work great in a "Mothers Day out" group where working moms chose to share the "burden" of daycare and all would benefit as a result.

> **NOTE TO READER:**
>
> Losing 4-5 days of pay a month, roughly 40 hours will cost you less than paying daily for daycare for a whole month. Work the numbers, you'll see. And….you'll benefit more if you have more than one child in your family. (Based on gross income)

Daycare cost is OUTRAGEOUS and I don't live in a town where daycare expenses are as high as they are in big cities. I can only imagine how hard we all work to give our money away to daycares that don't take the best care of our children. In return, our children get sick, and worse, ignored if they are a good and quiet baby. No thank you!

Whatever "daycare" option you decide to take, remember that your children come first. If you don't like a certain daycare……..

> **A NOTE ABOUT DAYCARE COSTS:**
>
> I told you earlier that daycare employee's salaries are slim to none yet above I am stating that daycare cost is very expensive. Unfortunately, most of the money that a daycare facility collects is not paid to the people who teach your children. Overhead eats up much of the funds. Since I do not own a daycare, I cannot comment on where the rest goes. However, I do know the excess funds do not end up in the teachers' pockets. Most daycare facilities do not even offer insurance to their employees (teachers) so it is a transient work force due to minimal pay and minimal benefits.

switch! Do not hesitate to pay the daycare application fee to a new daycare even if your child has only attended their current daycare facility for one month. Your child is WELL WORTH the small amount of money you are paying (again) to see that they are taken care of while away from your home and your heart during the day. Don't leave your children at daycare longer than 8-9 hours a day maximum. They need you and if you are old enough to have a child, then please be responsible enough to raise them on your own when you have the time after work.

CHAPTER 7
Breastfeeding and Pumping

I got out of the gym shower one morning and proceeded to my bench in the locker room where I dried off and got dressed for the day. I inspected my breasts and tucked them in my bra and felt of them to see if the milk had already let down (it usually does in the shower) and I suddenly caught a glimpse of my self in the mirror. "Do most people touch their breasts?" I begin to look around, "Was all that fondling necessary?" Or was I just so used to touching myself from feeding Nathaniel that I completely forgot the rest of America could be watching me and thinking, 'What on earth is she doing over there?'"

I can remember my sister's breasts being so big while breastfeeding that she literally had to lean over into her bra to get "them" (you could have named them they were so large) to fit in her bra and then she would arrange them, one at a time, as though they had their own separate personalities.

It is true that your breasts are the objects of someone's desire! And, it is not your husband's…..but your sweet little infant's. You will probably be pumping, squeezing and holding your breasts more in the next year than you will in your whole lifetime. It is crazy to think that we hardly ever touch ourselves except to apply lotion or maybe take a glimpse of ourselves unclothed in the mirror. But truly, it can be embarrassing to realize you are the only one in a

> **A NOTE ABOUT BREASTFEEDING:**
>
> Did you know that when most women begin breastfeeding it will stop menstruation and procreation for a period of 3-12 months? It is true that you do not have a period when breastfeeding (for most women, there are exceptions). You usually will not conceive during this period of time either. It's your body's way of taking its time to recover. However, we all hear of the horror story of a mother getting pregnant only a few months after her newborn's birth. So, be smart about your fertility, and be sure to ask for birth control at your six week post pregnancy check-up with your doctor. Micronor® is a birth control for breastfeeding mothers (generic brand is Camila®, there are several others). Breastfeeding birth control pills are only 96% effective when compared to normal birth control pills which are 99% effective to preventing pregnancy.
>
> ***BE SURE TO USE BACK-UP PROTECTION IF YOU ARE TAKING ANTIBIOTICS OF ANY SORT (especially penicillin derivatives). ANTIBIOTICS CAN CAUSE YOUR BIRTH CONTROL TO BE INEFFECTIVE, speaking from one who knows!!!!

room holding yourself to keep milk from leaking on your shirt while the rest of the world stares at you and thinks, "What is she doing!?"

On this note I would like to lead into returning back to work and your decision with pumping your breasts..........

Pumping the boobs:
To be or not to be? That is the question!

This is a strange and odious chore that we as mothers have to deal with at work if we want to keep breastfeeding when we return home to our children. Some mothers will choose to breastfeed only for the short time they are on maternity leave with their children. If that is your choice, feel great in knowing you have done your best to supply your child with the necessary antibodies to fight off illnesses that may "lurk in the dark." However, most of us choose to continue with breastfeeding in an effort to keep a bond with our newborn though we must be away from them while working. Obviously, we still get the satisfaction of knowing that our children's immune systems are gaining antibodies needed and your child is getting the "best of the best" that the world has to offer, which is your breast milk.

Again, this topic can be a touchy subject for husbands and wives. My ex-husband was a formula fed-bottle baby. Naturally, he is as strong and healthy as a horse, so he believes that bottle feeding is the way to go. I, on the other hand was breastfed, and have an immune system the size of a gnat. His answer to the question of which is the better option, 'breast or bottle fed babies,' is a simple one: obviously bottle fed children grow stronger, faster, and better since he did, right?

Wrong! Just because you breastfeed, there is no guarantee your child will be sniffle or cough free for his lifetime. Still, your breast milk does give your child a better chance against fighting sicknesses you may have dealt with in your lifetime that formulas cannot provide for your child. The antibodies that your body produced to fight off the flu last year, a kidney infection a year ago, or a bad cold the month before, will be passed on to your child through your breast milk. Breast milk is not a sure fire way to guarantee your child's good health, but it is a way to ensure that you are placing much needed nutrients and some antibodies in your baby. These antibodies may keep your child from getting sick in the future….and formula fed babies just don't get that benefit as of yet. Now that's food for thought!

So, how do you choose between breast and bottle?

You make the right choice for you and move on. Clearly, I am a mother who breastfeeds, so I will discuss pumping, breastfeeding, and my experience on both of those topics. However, I think feeding from the bottle with formula is an obvious and good choice for those mothers who do not feel comfortable with breastfeeding, or whose milk does not express after giving birth.

When Julia was born, I started to breastfeed immediately. I can remember one thing: My breasts almost fell off!

I have heard so much discussion from mothers who say they have tried to breastfeed and their milk wouldn't express two days after giving birth. *Let me explain a few things here:* Your infant was born with a little bit of extra fat for two reasons: 1) Infants

> **NOTE TO READER:**
>
> If your milk does not come in after giving birth and you desire to breastfeed, you can have a shot or take medicine to help your milk come down. Also, when breastfeeding, if your milk begins to wane naturally, you can increase your milk supply by taking medicine which will help you prolong your breastfeeding experience. This option is a good one for mothers who are losing their milk supply gradually. Remember that medications are only temporary (as long as you take the medicine) and not a permanent fix. Still, the 'drug produced' breastfeeding is better than giving up for some mothers who wish to give their child the best nutrients as well as having the breastfeeding experience for themselves.

> **PROBLEM:**
>
> Lots of mothers fear that because their baby doesn't appear to be "nourishing" her body (i.e. they don't see milk pouring out of their breast) that their baby will starve too death. They immediately give up breastfeeding proclaiming they don't have enough milk or that the milk won't come in and they convert to the bottle/formula, thereby not giving their body the "natural" chance to do what it can do for their child.

naturally sleep a lot the first few days after being born, therefore they have extra body fat to sustain them until they become more aroused; and 2) Milk "let down" does not happen instantaneously after giving birth! It takes time for a mother to begin milk production and learn the art of breastfeeding. Your milk will begin to come in within the first 24-72 hours after birthing your child. When your milk does come in, YOU WILL KNOW IT! Your breasts get really engorged and you will feel helpless trying to breastfeed your tiny little infant with this huge basketball sized breast full of milk. The infant may not even be able to get your nipple in its mouth because your breast is so full of milk. Prior to "let down," you may feel a burning sensation or heat come rushing to the nipple and top of your breast, and "bam!-" the milk is there. Until that point, you have colostrum (foremilk), the precursor to breast milk, which is full of antibodies and minerals. Some mothers don't even have lots of colostrum, they just have a few trickles for the first few days and then their milk comes in.

When Julia began eating during the first two days in the hospital, I felt as though I barely supplied her with any nourishment. This was in fact, natural! This was our time to get to know one another. The nurse would bring her to me every two hours and we would work on breastfeeding. I was so shy about getting a lactation consultant in the room with me. Julia's little head was bobbing all over the place trying to root in and find the "target." Finally, we would connect and it was all I could do to relax because of the pain associated with feeding her the first few days. The books say "relax, don't lean forward or in, bring the baby to you, etc." "Excuse me; this little person is chewing a part of my body off! I am going to do my best to maintain composure! If I lean in, struggle, hop all over the bed, and grit my teeth, I have done well enough for the first few times as long as I didn't hurt my infant in the process!"

> **CHECK YOURSELF OUT:**
>
> If either of your breasts becomes red, painful to touch, or feel engorged even after you just fed your child or pumped and you are having flu like symptoms with a fever: CALL YOUR DOCTOR! You probably have a common breast infection in your milk duct. Unfortunately this infection will not go away on its own, you must take prescription drugs to clear up the infection. Your breast may even look streaky or discolored with a red streak, and skin will be warm to the touch as the infection progresses.

Another myth:

The books say to feed on each breast for 20-30 minutes at a time. **THIS HAS <u>NEVER</u> <u>EVER</u> HAPPENED FOR ME**. My children have both breastfed just fine and not once has either of them fed for more than 15 minutes on each breast. Julia and Nathaniel's whole entire feeding lasted 20-25 minutes maximum. I used to say that my infants must be efficient little eaters. Now, I am finding more and more mothers say the same thing about their breastfeeding sessions with their children. **Why then do books insist on saying that it takes so much longer?** I was *feeling inadequate because I thought I wasn't giving my child enough nourishment.* Relish the pleasure and simplicity of feeding your child with the ease and convenience of breastfeeding and realize it doesn't take a long time to breastfeed *the right way.*

I used lanolin cream on my nipples for relief. I tried massaging my nipples. However, mostly I lay in bed and held those burning nipples until I cried, dreading the next feeding time. By week two, one nipple was cracked and in pain and the other was hanging on its last limb. "Can I do this anymore?" Could I go on!? I thought not! I thought if I had to feed her even just one more time, I would cave in on myself and dissolve away in to nothingness. I was in utter pain at the thought of that little mouth coming toward me again. Besides, I thought "She's not getting much milk now anyway, right?" Well, at the end of two weeks, I just about gave up breastfeeding. Then, a very strange thing occurred. My nipples just all of a sudden didn't hurt anymore. The crack healed up and started scabbing over and I was more

> **GOOD BUY TIP:**
>
> *"Secrets of the Baby Whisperer"* by Tracy Hogg (http://www.babywhisperer.com). An excellent book that I can't say enough about, with all sorts of tips from nursing your child to learning your babies cues of what they need when they cry. She goes over sleeping problems, crib issues, and methods for raising your child ("Why choose just one?"). I found this book well worth the money and would also recommend her second edition for toddlers. I read both books in about two days. Her books are fabulous and I can't say enough about how much her knowledge has helped me become a better mother. Losing Tracy to melanoma in 2004 was truly a loss for mothers all over the world. She wrote one final book before her death in 2004 for solving all your baby's problems.

relaxed. In fact, my nipples were kind of numb to the touch and I wasn't leaning in for each feeding (which again can cause you so much more effort and pain than it's worth, no wonder people quit before giving it a serious try). I began to relax. I began to feel my milk let down and know when it was time to feed Julia not only by her cues, but by my body's cues. I had tons of milk, I couldn't feed her enough. My breasts were staying engorged all the time!

The Pump:

After much debate, lots of breast pain, and aggravation, I bought a Pump in Style® top of the line breast pump from Medela, Inc. Instant relief! These pumps pull the milk out with ease. I found that even though it was a little rough on higher settings, I could turn it down and it would express my milk without a flinch of my body. How wonderful! Pumping at work does not have to be pure hell on your breasts.

Three of my friends bought **Pump in Style®** pumps from yard sales. *I was leery about doing that because I knew nothing about breast pumps and felt I would be contaminated from the previous owner's use of the pump.* Nonsense! All the pump does is supply you

> **BIG MISTAKE:**
> We waited until I went back to work to purchase a top of the line breast pump and I suffered through the first 2-3 months of breastfeeding with a hand me down hand held battery operated pump. <u>WHAT A DISASTER!</u> I spent hours at a time trying to get out the milk, and the pump pinched my nipple and made it hurt. Later, I splurged and bought a $40.00 pump sold at a local retail store. Still no relief! The box description made it sound as though the pump was as good as the expensive pumps. Really, it did nothing for me but cause more pain and gave less milk than a top of the line pump would have expressed.

with a motor to pull out the milk. The pump is cute and comes in a black bag that looks like a briefcase. You will have to buy new components (bottles, tubing for the hook up, and the breast shield to collect the milk) to pump with as these components you would not want to pass on to the next user. However, the pump is much cheaper if bought at a yard sale for around $40-$50, versus $200-$250 for a brand new pump (with components). You can buy pump components to replace the used parts at a medical service store. I recommend this pump to every working mother. Don't wait until after you have the baby to buy one.

I had been pumping successfully for a few months with the hand held battery operated pump, but wish someone would have told me to buy a good pump available from the very first day of my child's birth? Why?

You can begin pumping and help your milk come in as well as pump when your newborn infant is sleeping and your breasts are engorged with milk. You can also pump in between feedings because early on in your child's birth, you are producing so much more milk than your infant will eat. Most of us ignore that "full breast" feeling and just wait till the next feeding, but you shouldn't. You should pump that milk and store it up for a "rainy day." *Struggling through with my hand held battery operated pump, I had saved up about ten -4 ounce servings of breast milk. Six weeks after having given birth to Julia, I got very sick and was in the hospital. I was so thankful I had saved up the breast milk, but angry I had not purchased a better pump to express more milk. Julia ended up with a limited milk supply and I was faced with giving her formula at a very young age, when frankly, I didn't want to give her formula, ever (as I had to throw away my milk that I pumped while in the hospital because it had drugs in it from the medication I was taking)!*

My mom stepped in and came up with the ingenious idea to mix what little breast milk I had with formula. I was able to give Julia some essence of "me" in every bottle she ate. I thought that was a great idea since it was important to me that Julia remained breastfed and I recommend mixing formula with your pumped milk if you are a mother struggling with milk production. It took me forever to find the right formula for Julia. I was busy using all the samples of formula that I had received from the doctor's office and through the mail. *Have you ever tasted that stuff personally? It's nasty!* Try **Nestle Good Start** (milk based). This formula doesn't "smell" like some of the others and is a formula that I found Julia would actually tolerate on its own when my milk supply was short.

From the time I went back to work, I had to struggle with providing Julia enough breast milk, so finding a formula I could mix in with my breast milk on days I didn't produce enough milk was a good solution.

When you spend the whole weekend breastfeeding your child and return to work on Monday, you will pump more milk on Monday than any other week day. Breastfeeding naturally stimulates milk production and pumping is only second best. That's why feeding your infant from the breast during the work week in the mornings and at night is so important. I can't stress enough that there is absolutely nothing that can replace the suckling your child will do which releases chemicals in your brain telling your milk to "come on out!"

Still, many moms wait until they get that "let down" feeling to pull out the pump and start pumping whether at home or at work.

I did the same thing with Julia. Hhmmm! It never occurred to me that I could try pumping before I got the "let down" sensation in order to increase my milk supply. With Nathaniel, pumping before the "let down" feeling worked very well.

It's not you!

"What was I doing wrong?" Some of my best friends could pump up to 20 ounces a day (and if you are one of those mothers, God bless your mammary glands). I was pumping a meager 10 ounces a day on Monday, my highest milk producing day of the week. Frustrating! Well, after about 7 months of struggling, I called the lactation consultant. I knew there was a medication I could try to increase my milk supply.

It is called Reglan®. Reglan® (Metoclopramide) is a drug taken on a short-term basis for acid reflux, but one side effect is that it causes lactation (and in some cases, depression), or for breastfeeding mothers, an increase in lactation. [3] Yea! Hallelujah! *I took Reglan® and my milk was coming out again as it did when Julia was born.* The lactation consultant recommended doing a "tapering dose schedule" of Reglan®. The schedule was three pills a day for two weeks, two pills a day for two weeks, and then one pill a day for two weeks. Reglan® worked like a charm! However, I found that as soon as I was off the Reglan®, I was back to my regular old wimpy supply of milk. I had to be creative!

The following is an e-mail I sent to a girlfriend who was having problems with her milk supply. The e-mail explains tips and alternatives for prolonging your milk supply for your infant.

---

[3] Creative Impacts, Use of Reglan® to Increase Milk Supply, http://www.breastfeeding.org/articles/reglan.html

E-mail:

I know you have been told this a thousand times, but drink the absolute most amount of water you can. I know that I don't drink enough water (and I drink a lot) and water consumption has lots to do with milk production. Buy a big container of water and take it with you everyday, drink at least two containers of water daily (I use my hospital cup or an empty cranberry juice bottle from the store, about 64 fl. oz.). I used to hate drinking water until I discovered that distilled water tastes better than all the spring waters. Distilled water doesn't have all the funky minerals that the spring waters do. Try distilled water or filtered water from your refrigerator. You can freeze your water the night before, and leave it on your desk to thaw all day while drinking it bit by bit so that you always have fresh cold water (although some medical reports claim the plastic containers leach a toxic chemical out when frozen so do this at your own discretion).

Pump before your breasts "let down". A lot of times the "pumping action" will cause your milk to come in even though you don't realize it. I used to wait for "let down" before I would pump. Not anymore! Pumping before the "let down" feeling might help your milk come in more often. Increase your pumping even though you aren't producing milk in that volume. Remember, the more nursing you do over the weekend (hence, more feedings, i.e. pumping sessions simulated), the

> **BOTTOM LINE:**
>
> Remember there are no quick fixes, Reglan® is only temporary. You will need to implement some changes and be persistent in your quest to produce milk if you feel you would like to continue breastfeeding. Pumping is one of the most difficult jobs a mother has to do and it is so under appreciated. However, it comes with the benefits of knowing you are nurturing your child with the best nutrients possible.

more your breasts will try to produce milk. Even if you pump 5 minutes for 4-5 times a day and get nothing, your breasts will still try to produce more milk versus pumping for 2-3 times a day for 15 minutes at a time.

Massaging your breast: When your baby is breastfeeding and/or when you are pumping, take your breast in your hand (thumb on top) and grasp it like you were trying to squeeze a banana out of the peel. Take your thumb and press gently but firmly from the top of your breast down. Repeat this over and over again while pumping or feeding. You can also massage in a circular motion with your finger tips, again from the veins/vessels running from the top of your breast, down toward the nipple and around in a circular motion. Even after you think the milk is "gone" if you start to massage your breasts in the above mentioned manner, you'll get a few extra squirts (hey, every drop counts!).

Getting more sleep and having less stress: More sleep and less stress WILL make a difference. Don't stress so much about it, and don't forget to mix your breast milk in with the formula to help curb the formula taste.

Don't worry, the Reglan® will kick in: The key is that while the meds are working, be sure to save up all the milk you can (freeze, pump extra at home when your baby doesn't need it and is sleeping. You could be working to save up that milk, even if it's an ounce!) Don't forget to drink your water even though you are on Reglan®, and treat it as though after the Reglan® ends you will still need to be implementing the above notes. Once something is working, there is a tendency to slack off. Don't! Remember Reglan® is only temporary.

Be leery of the teas and herbs: I read some books that say the mother's consumption of the wrong herbs may possibly harm your infant's liver.

Although some teas in small amounts are okay to try, do some research to find out the pros and cons of teas and herbs.

I would start Friday afternoons after work, feeding my babies naturally from the breast. When I felt let down, I would try to feed Nate off of one breast completely. If he seemed satisfied, I pumped the other breast for storage. If not, I fed him off the other breast and then waited for next time. I broke his feedings up to where I didn't wait for him to get hungry; I fed him about every 2-4 hours. Kurk said I was always shoving my breast in his mouth! But hey, I gotta do something to keep the milk going, and Nate didn't mind a bit. These smaller feeding sessions helped me keep producing ample milk and gave me an opportunity to produce more milk rather than have less feeding sessions and less milk. There is nothing like having your baby breastfeed, it helps that milk come down so much more than pumping. AND, don't forget to have a picture of your child with you at work.

NOTE TO READER:

It is natural for your breast milk production to drop off around 4-5 months after the baby is born. Pumping mothers notice this problem and feel like something is horribly wrong because they aren't collecting as many milk bottles as they were just a few weeks ago (mothers who exclusively breastfeed don't even realize their milk supply naturally weans because they do not measure their milk supply). Your body is designed to produce the precise amount of milk needed for your child, and when your child's need for maximum nourishment is required, maximum breast milk is produced. Likewise, when your child needs less breast milk, your body produces less breast milk. Some of us have a problem with creating ample milk supply from the start of our child's birth. But….for the most part, you should have plenty of milk for you baby until you choose to stop breastfeeding or your baby decides to wean himself.

If you can call wherever she/he is staying during the day and listen to your child talk, sometimes that will make your milk come down too (just hearing your infant's cry or talking about her can do that).

Last, try breastfeeding lying down (on your side) with your infant beside you on the bed. I found that this was the most relaxing way to feed Nate (I did this with Julia too). Breastfeeding produces natural chemicals to help the mom sleep, so take a nap while feeding during the day (on the weekends or whenever you feed him/her) and that will help you relax even more.

Kurk and I both were highly opposed to bringing Julia to bed with us when we had her, but I would bring her to bed with me when she would wake during the night in her crib and feed her on and off during the night switching sides while sleeping in our bed. So she would start off sleeping in her crib, and then around 1-3A.M., I would go get her when she would wake crying to feed and bring her to bed with me for the rest of the night. You must be careful not to roll over on your baby while sleeping, but this option of feeding will help too.

With Nate, I brought him to bed with us and Kurk didn't mind a bit. It was so much easier for me rather than getting up and down a million times a night. The 'ups and downs' at night are enough to stress anyone out and make them tired for work the next day.

Nate slept in his crib for about 5-6 hours a night. When he got older and I didn't have to worry about feeding him throughout the evening, then I worked on acclimating him to his crib for the 12 hour sleeping period.

Last, you can sneak a feeding in while your infant is sleeping. Feed your baby just before you put her down for her night's sleep. Then, right before you go to bed (2-3 hours should have passed since you put your baby to sleep) just pick her up out of her crib, sit in the rocker or lie on the bed, and feed her again. Don't wake her, simply pry open her mouth, pop in your boob, and you'll see it's your child's natural reaction to suckle. She will be eating and you will find you can keep her asleep and in her crib that much longer during the night instead of her waking up just a few hours after you lie down for the night.[4]

> **TIP:**
>
> Motherlove Herbal Company specializes in products to "pump up" your milk supply. I have not used these herbal supplements and am not necessarily suggesting there use. However, I felt inclined to add the website (www.motherlove.com) for those nursing moms who are interested in trying an herbal supplement that may help their milk supply.

Some lactation help:

There are some herbs such as mint, sage and parsley which might cause your milk supply to decrease. You should definitely avoid these herbs when trying to nurse your child. However, they are safe to use when you begin to wean your baby (Refer to Breast Milk Interactions Charts website below).[5]

Duh! I thought I was avoiding mint, sage and parsley and then one day I realized I use mint flavored ChapStick®! I am sure that has an effect too, so keep all non-food products consisting of these plants

---

4 Hogg, Tracy, with Blau, M., *Secrets of the Baby Whisperer*, New York Times, 2001, http://www.babywhisperer.com
5 BabyCenter, L.L.C., Breast Milk Interactions Charts, 1997-2003, http://www.babycenter.com/general/8788.html.

from ingestion or absorption as well (don't forget shampoos and body washes too!).

Where, 'Oh where do the pumping girls go?

I have had three different friends recently ask me where I went to pump when I returned to work (what office or location). I strongly suggest that you talk about this issue with your boss before having your baby. Therefore, when you go back to work after maternity leave, you and your boss will both know what to expect when it comes to your pumping time.

The La Leche League International

The La Leche League International has web pages (http://www.lalecheleague.org/organization) and links about your rights as a "pumping mother" and your rights in the work place. *Did you know breastfeeding in public used to be a federal offense?* Now you can breast feed legally in public. I drive my mother crazy with this breastfeeding conundrum. I guess I was more modest before having Julia, but now that I have Nathaniel, I will pretty much whip it out anywhere if he gets hungry. The "whipping out of my breast" is not what mother has the issue with, rather, it is the "hook up of baby to nipple" that causes my mother much duress. I find that when "hooking up" and having my shoulder draped with a blanket, I end up dropping the blanket (which I DO NOT want touching the store floor, buggy, or anything unsanitary) and everyone sees my "business" anyway. I have found if I turn the opposite way of most of the isle traffic, or either go in to a corner of the store, I can "hook up" without much complication or eyes watching and then I can drape (with my mothers assistance) making it much easier to feed while in transit. *I must make a personal note that if you get really good at it, you can carry your baby with your shirt just covering the edge of their face while they are eating and no one would even know you are breastfeeding draped or not, they would just think the infant was sleeping in your arms.*

--So back to the issues of pumping at work: There are laws being put in front of congress to explore mandatory breaks during the work week to allow a mother to pump and store breast milk. You should discuss "break issues" for pumping with your boss well in advance of returning to work. Most of the time, your boss should be very accommodating. My bosses have let me pump in my office without any trouble. My first pumping experience at work was one where I was housed in a "cubby/cubical" type desk without a private door. I took a linen sheet to work and clipped it up with some binder clips and posted a note that said "Do not enter when sheet is up." Sure you could here the pump running, but nobody really knew what was going on behind the curtain except me. As long as you are discreet, no one will even care anyway. My second time around, I had an office with shutting doors. Frequently, I would find that the doors were being opened so I could help others and answer questions. I was sure to face my back to the door so that no one would see that I was busy pumping. I have even had people standing right next to me, deep in conversation and suddenly say, "What is that noise I hear?" Since the pump looks like a briefcase, they were clueless that I was pumping right before their very eyes. The facial expressions I would get from people when they realized I was pumping while they were standing there was priceless! However, I figured I had to do what I had to do whether or not they were in my office. I had said if the door is shut then don't come in because I was pumping. Otherwise, if the door was open, they should know I'm ready for "business."

Most work places do have a "nurse's station" or break room that can be set up for breastfeeding/pumping mothers. I have several friends who do go to the nurse's station for their own comfort and feeling of privacy to pump their breast milk. For me, I saw pumping as a very natural process. I did want my privacy; however, I was not going to walk two floors up with all my belongings each time to do a task that literally took 10 minutes if everyone left me alone. That's my opinion, like it, or pump it! Ha!

Disinfecting bottles and nipples: How much is too much?

When I first got my breast pump, I read all the instructions. I had to boil this and replace that and take all the parts apart and do this after every pump session. Okay, big clue here gals: I don't have time to boil, scrub and wash everything! I work full time, so I need something fast and handy.

Did you know that the nearest thing to an autoclave (which they use to sterilize the tools in your dentist's office) sits in your very household and you probably use it everyday? It is a dishwasher. Though dishwashers do not have the pressure of cleaning that an autoclave has, they are capable of supplying us with two very important items: HEAT and BLEACH. That's right folks! You can clean your pump equipment in your dishwasher. If you don't have a dishwasher, get one! You can buy a dishwasher that hooks up to your sink if you can't afford the permanent models. You can even buy small ones now that plug into the wall and sit countertop on your kitchen counter space. I take the pump pieces, pull them apart, and throw them right into the top basket in my dishwasher (you know, the cool little baskets for the dishwashers that every new parent gets at their baby showers). I add the detergent (which should have bleach in it), turn it on, and go. That's it.

I am not suggesting that washing the pump parts in the dishwasher in any way sterilizes as thoroughly as boiling water. Furthermore, if you feel more comfortable boiling things, by all means, do so! For me, it was easier to place all the items in the dishwasher and move on. To this day, I wash Justin's pacifiers in the dishwasher. When the latex gets "sticky" or the silicone wears out, I simply throw them away and buy more.

Bleach is awesome and can kill even the strongest of diseases if used appropriately. However, bleach is toxic, so unless you can make a diluted concentration of bleach, I would not recommend using pure bleach to clean things in the sink. That's why I like detergents and soaps that contain bleach because they already have the right amount formulated in for you.

Nipples and pacifiers:

I have known several people (including myself) who have had the dilemma of getting a newborn to take to a bottle after the mom returns to work. Quite often the new mothers do not start experimenting with the bottle until a few days before going back to work. Taking a few days to research the kind of nipple and pacifier your child will like is something I strongly recommend you do before the "going back to work" day draws near.

Every infant is particular in their own way and will not necessarily use the same nipple or bottle as their brother or sister. Here's the trick to finding which nipple your child will like best:

First, start with the nipple that fits your breast pump storage bottles and holds only a few ounces (most likely around 4 ounces) in each bottle. There are silicon nipples, latex nipples, fast flow, slow flow, stage 1, stage 2 nipples, etc. A pack of nipples only cost about $1.50. I recommend first buying storage bottles for your breast milk (**Evenflo** makes these and sells them at retail stores in packs of four for about $4.00). Then, buy several different types of nipples and try one set at a time. Connect the nipple directly to the milk storage bottle for an easy conversion to a feeding bottle. If your baby doesn't like that nipple, throw all from that package out but one and try the next set of nipples. Try each nipple type until your infant finds one he likes and also doesn't choke on the milk flow (if you find you have to sit your infant upright to keep from choking on the milk, try a slow flow or a stage 1 nipple instead). If all nipple types are exhausted, then you must start trying different types of bottles with specialized nipples, made specifically for the bottle and sold as a pack. Borrowing bottles from a friend to just "try out" on your child is a perfect option. Most likely the first bottle you buy will not be the one your child will like (unless you have the luck of the Irish!).

Nathaniel did not like any of the nipples that fit the breast milk storage bottles. I remembered my sister had bought me some bottles (in the sale rack) at a retail

> **NOTE TO READER:**
>
> Don't forget to move up to Stage 2 or medium to high flow nipples as your child grows. If your child stops taking the bottle, one reason may be that it is too much work for him to get the milk out of the nipple.

store. I opened them up, threw them in the dishwasher, and tried them the next day. Ta-Da! He loved them and they worked perfectly. They are from the **Playtex® Nurser** series. The bottom of the bottle actually unscrews, thus making cleaning the bottle a breeze. The nipple is shaped wider, like a breast at the top, to simulate that of regular breastfeeding. I love these bottles and understand why Nathaniel thought they were so wonderful! He used the Stage 1 flow nipple with this bottle. Without this bottle, he was choking on his milk because the flow was too fast, but now he can drink with the comfort that he won't choke.

I never really wanted to store my breast milk in bags, it just seemed messy to me. However, I did try it. They bags toppled over and didn't stand upright while freezing in the freezer. I also had a hard time thawing the bags when the time came to use them in a bottle since I did not use the bottles with the disposable inserts with Julia. **Don't forget that you can use breast milk for only a short amount of time after thawed from the freezer (usually it is a one time use/warming within a 24 hour period from the time thawed).** Also, formula is only good for a limited period of time so be sure to read the enclosures that come with your milk storage bottles as well as the formula instructions for storage and long term preservation conditions.[6]

Bye, bye breast feeding, Hello… screwed up cycles!

This bit of text is totally uncorroborated from the medical experts, but I had to include it because I am finding more and more women

---

[6] Nemours Foundation, Kid's Health® for parents, Breastfeeding FAQs: Safely Storing Breast Milk, http://kidshealth.org/parent/growth/feeding/breastfeed_storing.html

experience these problems. One or two months after you finish breastfeeding you should start having periods again. At the initial onset of your first period, you will find nothing to be abnormal. However, for most of us, that soon changes. If you begin to experience a very heavy period every other week, this is in fact a normal process in my own personal experiences.

When my menstrual cycles began again after I stopped breastfeeding Julia, I freaked out due to the frequency of bleeding. What was wrong with my body??

I was told that changing birth control pills would control the "break through bleeding" occurring every other week and lasting for a week each time. As was explained to me, the birth control pills were no longer effective for my body as they once were. This "answer" for the excessive bleeding when your period starts back seems to be the general consensus among many doctors. However, I believe their consensus to be untrue. In fact, I think that having this "break through bleeding" or period every few weeks for the first 1-3 months after your period resumes is normal in order to get your system acclimated again with the natural ebb and flow of menstruation.

After Julia stopped breastfeeding and I started having problems with bleeding frequency, I tried switching birth control pills twice by my doctor's advice. The "break through bleeding" didn't stop until I had tried about 3 different pills. The time frame between switching my pills was about 1-3 months after I started menstruation. Based on this hunch, I stuck with the same birth control pill that I used while breastfeeding Nathaniel the second time around. As I suspected, I started having a period every other week without any birth control pill switching at all. After about 6 weeks, my normal cycle returned.

I usually have a 28-29 day cycle, and I found that I soon returned to the very same cycle without having done all the birth control switching I did with Julia to try and stop the break through bleeding.

Conclusion: When you resume having periods, your body will naturally fluctuate with a period every few weeks during the first 1-3 months until it finds your body rhythm and cycle again and then you will return to your regular monthly cycle.

I have since spoken with many friends who have experienced these same problems. I implore you to try sticking to the same birth control for 1-3 months before switching in an effort to reduce "break through bleeding."

> When you change birth control pills, you can experience break through bleeding, mood swings and depression. Additionally, birth control pills you've taken for years prior to conception may no longer work with your body's chemistry. I personally experienced frustration, seething anger and hot flashes when switching birth controls. After doing some research, I realized it was the birth control pill causing the mental stress. While trying to avoid break through bleeding I ended up causing mental aggravation, now there's a trade off (not!). If you have uncontrollable mood swings, mental anguish, or any symptoms of anger, you may want to consider researching your birth control pill a little more carefully with your doctor (or on-line, look for what others are saying about their experiences with your brand of birth control. Usually message boards on-line will give you a clue as to how your birth control pill is performing for other women around the world).

CHAPTER 8
Best Buys, Good Ideas and Pass em' On!

Have you ever wondered where your friend got the coolest car seat, the latest and greatest learning tool, or the best buy on an item for their child? I'm not sure why we don't share these tips with others. Are we in a hurry to "out-do" the other mothers and make them look bad? Sometimes things that may seem so "common sense" to you may totally pass by another person who has yet to think of such an easy and simple solution. I have taken the liberty of including some very common sense ideas as well as some good buys and must haves that have helped me keep my children safe and comfortable.

The first magazine I have to brag about is **One Step Ahead (Onestepahead.com)**. This magazine has a lot of the neat and cool inventions that all the "savvy shopping" mothers have. Their prices are reasonable. I can't say enough about this magazine and what it does for many mothers out there, myself included. I have bought several items from this company and each time I have been quite pleased with the item purchased.

Diaper Sense/Scents:

I was walking in to Julia's sitter's house one day and noticed that there was a stinky diaper on the porch wrapped in a plastic grocery bag. At first, I thought the diaper on the porch was rude, but then I realized her idea was ingenious! The Diaper Genie does a great job for young babies, but once your child starts to eat real solid foods, the consistency and the smell of the end result is not too pleasing to the nose, especially to the one who has to change the diapers. Needless to say, there isn't a trash can or diaper container no matter how well-made that won't allow the smell of this "aromatic little cloud" to seep all over the house. I added a twist, literally, and decided to do one thing more with the grocery bag. I take the bag, drop the diaper in, twist the bag as close to the diaper as possible, and turn the bag inside out on itself in order to wrap the diaper twice. Then, I use the handles of the bag to tie it tight and close to the diaper. Now, this isn't seal proof, but it does cut down on the smell, more so than just a knotted regular bag. All the help we can get in this department, the better!

Changing tables:

Some parents go through the expense of buying a whole changing table. Why not use the top of a low sitting dresser with a foam changing table on top of it? Now days you can get a terry cloth covering tailored to fit the changing table at your local wholesale store. They are wonderful! You can also buy these little washable "absorbance" pads that I place right underneath the area where my children's bottoms will be on the table, that way if I get something on the table, I don't have to wash the whole terry cloth cover every single time.

Bed Rails:

I could not find a bed rail for Julia's bed that I really liked. Most are made of plastic or mesh and are too short for the length of the bed. Others are down right hard to let up and down when getting in and out of the bed. **One Step Ahead** magazine has a bed rail that is out of sight fabulous. Although a bit pricey (at about $40.00) it is longer than any other bed rail I've seen. It is made of mesh and drops down and lifts up easily enough for Julia to get in and out of her bed. I have enjoyed this buy tremendously and think it was well worth the money.

eBay® buys:

I almost hate to mention this one because I am afraid of the competition I will get by mentioning this (let the bidding begin!). However, the internet auction house, eBay® is a WONDERFUL tool for purchasing items you need and want safely and without much risk. eBay® has so many baby items! In fact, almost anything you can think of you can buy on eBay®. I even buy my makeup from eBay® because it is so much cheaper and easier than going across town to the mall. It is delivered right to my front door! You would be surprised how wonderful and easy eBay® is to use. Try eBay®, but be sure to check out feed back for each seller to make sure you aren't buying from someone who tends to have negative feedback.

> **NOTE TO READER:**
>
> eBay® is a huge community with its own quirks and laws which define its users. Be sure to understand the rules and work within the confines of eBay.

Book Clubs:

I can't tell you how valuable buying books for your children at a young age can be. Kurk and I started purchasing books for Julia when she was an infant. First we bought the **Sesame Street ABC's** book set (**Reader Digest Young Families, Inc.** at http://www.rd.com/rdyf/splash.html). This book set is still one of my favorites because you can read them (each book represents a letter of the alphabet), you can put them together like a puzzle (which is on the back of each book cover) and you can hook them together in a line like a train. This book set also includes a floor mat for matching the books up on the puzzle, picture, number and alphabet flash cards and parent's newsletters. This set of books though a little pricey, can be easily purchased for less on eBay® if you are internet friendly.

As your children grow, you can try the Disney book series (purchased from Scholastic at http://www.scholastic.com). We bought enough books to fill the little paper book holder supplied with the books. I enjoyed this book series and found that although a little boring for me at times, Julia loved the simple pictures and simple words. The books talk about different things such as manners, objects, and routines.

> **BOTTOM LINE:**
>
> All book clubs are great, you can find a lot of them on line and if you sign up you usually get a few books free to try out and keep along with some other free items (like posters and book bags for joining). I highly recommend joining a book club, but be sure that when you have plenty of books from each series, to cancel your membership, or else the books will keep coming.

We are now into the Nick Jr. series of books (also with Scholastic) which I find very enjoyable, but some of the content is rather long to read. I do enjoy the artwork and the story lines and would refer this series to anyone.

Discount Stores (Dollar Stores):

When dollar stores first became popular, they sold a lot of junk worth about what they implied, a dollar. I hadn't stepped in a dollar store in years until my mom convinced me (dragged me) to go to a store one day. They have such a variety of things in dollar stores now days. It really is worth a separate trip to peek through the doors before shopping at your favorite super store. I was surprised to find grocery list pads, nail clippers, stationary and thank you notes, wrapping paper, tissue paper for presents, and birthday cards, all for a dollar each. They also have little travel pack size toys to choose from which I find so much easier to give to a two year old than the big versions you would buy at another store. For example, I was buying **Play-Doh™ (Hasbro at:** http://www.hasbro.com/playdoh) in the regular sized containers but Julia was making such a mess and we would argue about throwing some of it away after play time. Then, I found the small travel pack size at the Dollar Store and it was so convenient to use and easy to throw away and buy another pack when it dries out or the colors get mixed together. If you haven't been to a dollar store lately, you should reconsider, and if you are a grandmother, do the right thing and drag your daughters there kicking and screaming like mine did. Your daughters won't be sorry and will thank you as usual!

Pictures of the "youngin's"

Quality vs. Quantity: This is a tough topic to talk about because I have not had the experience of waiting thirty years to pull out my children's pictures from their younger years only to find they have faded and bleached out over time. We all have access to digital cameras now (love them!!!!). 'Scrap booking' moms out there probably know the best way to preserve an image in an album. Still, where is the best place to get your pictures taken and developed professionally? Most moms I know go to the discount photo studios and get their children's pictures made. Some mothers like to take their child every month in their first year of life to have a photo taken to show age progression of the child. However, I chose the 1 month, 3 month, 6 month, 9 month and 12 month ages (and then every 6 months there after) to have my children's photos made professionally. Photos are so expensive and you really must take advantage of the newest promotion each studio has to get the most for your money.

> **WORD OF CAUTION:**
>
> Some photo studios at discount prices give lots of pictures, but the preservatives on the photo (that cover the picture itself) do not last very long. Therefore, you may have great pictures now, but in 30 years, they may be faded and yellowed out. Be sure to pick a studio which preserves their pictures so you can enjoy your memories a lifetime. These studios may charge a bit more, but I believe in this case quality, not quantity is a must!

Olan Mills (http://www.olanmills.com) is a photo studio that used to make appointments for both sitting and pick up times with your photos. Olan Mills has revolutionized its photo taking process. No longer do you have the long appointment waits, although you can make an appointment, you can also "walk in" and get served on a first come first serve basis. Most professional studios have switched to digital technology, so there is no more waiting for your proofs to arrive. The companies let you pick your images on screen and you pay in advance for your promotional package right after photos are taken.

> **BIG FAT FLAG:**
>
> Photo companies do have a master plan! Remember they take at least six photos at every sitting, and your coupon only applies to the first photo they take in that sitting session. So, make sure your first pose is the exact pose you want so that you won't be tempted to buy the whole package each time you go to the portrait studio. Splurge and use your Super Saver Plan to buy the whole packages when every family member is included in the pictures.

What I do is buy the package set with a coupon each time (plus S&H) and then I buy one or two sheets separately. Although buying sheets separately can be expensive, it keeps me from purchasing everything on the table. Also, I always join their Super Saver Plan for a small fee (it used to be called the Watch Me Grow plan) and can get every picture of my children at whatever discount promotion they are offering for that year. I am always sure to print out the current web coupon which often times is a bit cheaper than the one in the local Sunday newspaper.

Bras & Tank tops:

Nursing bras are really a pain! However, they are a necessary evil for most of us new moms. The only bras I have really felt comfortable in have the front snap which enables easy release of the bra cup for nursing and cotton material for comfort. A good nursing bra cost about $18.00, and is usually well worth the money. I purchased mine from **Motherhood** (http://www.motherhood.com). Every bra I've ever owned that had an under wire (and this one does as well), eventually gave way on the end with the under wire popping out of the material on the side. My last bra also had the wire issue, however, my mom came up with an ingenious way to sew the wire back in so that it doesn't pop out again. Cutting a thick piece of cotton fabric half the length of your pinky finger and sewing it on top of the area where the wire pops out allows extra coverage to make sure that wire stays put. Be sure to place the extra fabric over the end of the area where the wire keeps popping out and sew it around the edges. This is a full-proof way to keep those under wires, well, under!

I found that buying cheap tank tops or tube tops sold during the summer at retail stores seem to be the best answer for sleeping at night and dealing with breastfeeding issues. How many times have you gone to bed in your granny panties and your ugly nursing bra (with the line across the middle, yucky, throw those away!) feeling like an unattractive mess. Wearing a tube top not only gives you ease of feeding your infant at night but also allows you a bit more comfort while sleeping. And, you don't have to look so much like a grandma in your underwear. I even used nursing pads for my milk leakage with the tube tops and it worked well. I would just remove the pad while feeding my child and then place it back in when done. No arranging to make everything line up in a bra before snapping it back, who needs that at 1 A.M. in the morning?!

Waking up in the night:

Does your child (infant and even your 2 year old toddler) wake up in the night for no reason at all?

They might be cold. I have noticed even during summer months (when the house seemed comfortable to me) that Julia would wake up during the night. I started putting a one piece pajama zip suit (with feet/stockings) on her and she began sleeping through the night immediately.

Be sure to cover your infant's head at night with a cap to retain warmth and remember some babies like to feel the weight of a blanket touching them. **A blanket can smother a child, so use extreme caution.** *With Julia, I didn't use any blankets because I was terrified of suffocation. With Nathaniel, I used blankets regularly and kept a close eye on him.*

Baby gates and door locks:

Have you ever awakened in the middle of the night to find your two year old cruising through the house? That is such and uncomfortable feeling and you wonder what other sort of trouble your little one might get into if you are fast asleep at night. Thank goodness for the invention of baby gates. They are available in every baby magazine and discount store. However, you have to be smart with baby gates because if your child becomes successful even once at climbing over, then the gate will be useless. If you don't set boundaries, the baby gate will not be useful and you will have to devise another method (although my mom suggested trying one baby gate mounted right above the lower gate to keep them from climbing over, now that's sneaky!).

One of my girlfriends was having just such trouble, (her son had learned to climb over the gate) so she decided to turn the doorknob handle to his bedroom inside out. She then locked him in his room at night so that she could be sure that he did not get into trouble in the house. Suffice it to say that she did have a baby monitor in the room so that she could hear (and see on some monitors) what was going on in the room while she wasn't in there. I think this is a safe, easy and effective remedy to keeping a determined night owl in there room at night. Kudos to this parent for thinking this one up!

A CHEAP FIX:

Instead of baby proofing items the retail stores try to sell, why not try a cheaper method to safe guard your child from common dangerous household items? For example, a simple rubber band can be wrapped around door knobs instead of using the knob locks the baby proof manufacturers sell. Shutting the bathroom door saves you the worry of buying a toilet bar that locks the lid down (to ensure your child doesn't drown). Temporarily removing glass tables from the living room allows your infant hassle free walking space with no purchasing of cushiony pads to wrap that glass table in. Let's face it; the table suddenly doesn't look so fashion conscientious once doctored up with baby proof stuff anyway.

Parent Pages:

Most websites these days have "Parenthood Pages" that parents can subscribe to for a free monthly newsletter about many topics. For example, Gerber™ (http://www.gerber.com/home) and Pampers™ (http://us.pampers.com/en_US/home/home.jsp;jsessionid=DI1N5NR3WXNELQFIAJ0X0NQ) both have mail flyers and email web pages to keep you up to date on what your child should be doing at their age. I suggest you look carefully through your hospital baby bag and fill out the ads you get for free magazine subscriptions to Baby Talk, Pampers and Gerber. The more information you can get your hands on, the better. If you already know the answers, you can simply recycle the magazine when it comes in the mail.

Pass em' On!

Why in the world does every mother have to have a new one of everything before the baby is born?

This was my attitude before I had Julia. I felt everything had to be in its own fresh little wrapper or box waiting for me to unwrap, wash and proclaim that it was new and JUST for Julia in order to feel good about having it.

Granted, there are some items you will want brand new and just for your child: say for example their first little outfit you bring them home in from the hospital, their first rubber ducky, pacifier, or bath towel. But, wait about 6 months and you'll be screaming for any hand me down you can get your hands on, especially if the money to pay for these items is coming out of your pocket.

I was trying to be so pristine and careful not to accept anything I thought wouldn't be good enough for my child while I was pregnant with my firstborn. Molly kept trying to slough off all of this USED stuff and I just wouldn't have a thing to do with it. I did take the used bassinet, bouncer seat and Johnny jump up, but other than that, I bought a lot of things new. I hesitantly took pregnancy clothes, old bottles, baby clothes, towels, washcloths, a breastfeeding pillow and diaper pails for fear of hurting her feelings.

Until……

I was about to give birth to Julia and having already had all my showers, noticed Julia's closet was half-empty and barely contained any clothes. I went down stairs to view what I had in the way of used infant clothes. Wow! What a surprise! I had tons! I had previously sold all of the pregnancy clothes at a yard sale a few years back because the colors and styles weren't for me (big mistake, I was praying for anything to wear that fit and looked half way decent 5 months in to my pregnancy). At least I had learned from my yard sale experience to hold on to the infant clothes. Hey, what's the old saying, "If you fool me once shame on you, fool me twice, shame on me!" I took all the clothes and washed them immediately and got them ready for use. My sister took good care of all of the infant clothes and had stored most of them in crates for storage. Though she had not separated them into "age and sex" piles for use, I found this way of passing on clothes was a wonderful idea. Molly had given me boys and girls clothes (she now had two children, a girl and a boy). I didn't need the boy's clothes right away because I was having a little girl. So, I loaned the whole crate of boy's clothes to a friend of mine who was due a few days before me and was to have a little boy. She would use the clothes in the crate, and when her son would outgrow them, she'd throw them back in the crate and return them to me. I would bring the next stage (age range) of clothes to her and we would repeat the process!

No matter the size, put em' on:

When you are a first time parent, it doesn't dawn on you that the labels on the baby clothing may be inaccurate.

When Julia was a baby, I read the label to all her baby clothes, if it didn't say "newborn" or "0-3 months," I simply didn't try it on her. Then, I realized there were a ton of clothes in the closet she was going to miss wearing because they weren't "exactly" the right size for the season we were in. My sister said, "Oh, no, no! Try on everything, and if it doesn't fit exactly, roll the sleeves up or the pants legs up! Don't miss a chance to dress your baby in something that could have good wear because it doesn't fit perfectly." Then, I started reading clothing labels and trying on things more carefully, only to realize that half the time the labels aren't correct. Labels could say something is a 12 month's outfit, but your 6 month old baby may be wearing the "bigger" size with no problem. Never go by the label. Instead, be sure to try on everything. If it is a bit too big, just roll it up!

What a wonderful way to get a lot of use out of clothes that our children wear for such a brief period of time. But hey, it doesn't stop there. Don't forget about baby swings, cribs, excer-saucers, bottles, etc. Everything you can think of can be passed on from child to child. Just think, your child could be like Oprah, wearing each outfit only once because she has such a large inventory of clothes to choose from. Hey, and don't forget someone else's left over diaper stock (clean of course!). Their outgrown diaper sizes become your treasure.

I am pleased that I have started thinking it is necessary to do everything you can to save money and still get some nice looking and useful material goods for your children. Don't be shy about asking to buy something at a yard sale for a buck! Some people will literally give away items at the end of a yard sale. Don't forget to always stick to your instinct.

Speaking of.......

While we are on the topic of clothes and swapping them out, I want to talk to you a little about your own personal wardrobe. Are you the person who has three different sizes of clothing in your closet hogging up valuable rack room that you could be using with clothes you've got stuffed in your drawers of your dressers? I know for women it is important to keep clothes of varying sizes around since our bodies' cycle through different stages in life (having babies, being out of shape, being in shape, etc.). Instead of having an array of clothes sizes in your closet, take the ones you cannot wear right now and pack them in a crate and store them in the basement or attic. Then, as the seasons change, you can pick your crate labeled "Size 12, Winter" or "Size 10, Summer" and you have a whole new wardrobe awaiting you. You can also keep your husband from saying that you have a whole closet full of clothes yet you have nothing to wear. Truth is you do have a closet full of clothes you can't wear.......for now! But not forever. Be clothes smart and make space for the things you need now. Pulling out a few items that are too small and hanging them facing out so you can see them (maybe your favorite summer size 10 shorts outfit) can be a way to encourage yourself to continue to work toward that weight loss goal you are striving to reach. Stay strong my friend, you can do it!

CHAPTER 9
When They're Sick!

Colic, fevers, urinary tract infections, skin funkiness and more:

I remember the first time Julia was sick: it was such a scary event for a new parent like me. I had dropped by a friend's work place to let her see my new five week old baby. We visited and talked together, all the while she was holding my child in her arms. When I went to take Julia from her, I noticed immediately that her back was screaming hot. Her first fever! And, a high one at that: It ranged from 101°F to 103°F at its highest. I was frantic, miserable. Julia's pediatrician called us to the emergency room and we met him there to find a barrage of tests ready for her. We were very scared and nervous. She had blood drawn, medicine administered and a catheter which took urine to test for infection. After two long days of waiting, it was apparent from the urine culture that she had a urinary tract infection. We were prescribed the correct medicine and the problem went away.

Now all this sounds very easy and straight forward, but in reality, going to the doctor's office, getting a straight answer and finding a cure for "what ails" your child can be a very bumpy ride from beginning to end.

Try to see it from a doctor's point of view:

First let me say that every doctor who is a pediatrician should and probably does love children deeply. Whether or not they have children is insignificant. Rather, their ability to show love and care for your child, as well as having the knowledge to answer your questions and provide the proper health care when needed are the most important characteristics of your child's pediatrician and for your piece of mind.

One thing I often hear from parents is that the doctors don't know what they are doing, that they gave the child the wrong medicine, wrong dose, or sent the patient home no better off than when they arrived in the doctor's office (minus the cash for the office visit let's not forget).

It is VERY HARD in this day and age to diagnose illnesses. Imagine how difficult it can be for you to decide sometimes if your child, who you know very well, should really go to the doctor because they are acting a "little off" that day. It is equally if not more difficult for a doctor to assess your child's illness within a 15 minute time frame. This amount of time is usually the average time you see the pediatrician with your child, if not less once in the patient room, unless they are seriously ill. Doctors have very little time to see you and your child, so that time needs to be quality time. You need to have your questions ready, your mind clear on what symptoms you have witnessed, and your thoughts or ideas about what you think this illness might be so that you can contribute to a diagnosis. Doctors rely on this information. When we as parents don't give the doctors the background information, well, it leaves them guessing at a diagnosis.

You should know that a doctor would love nothing more than to send you home with a prescription each and every time you came to the office. If not so much that the prescription was needed, but in fact to ease your mind as a parent that your trip was worth the effort and that you didn't go home empty handed with no hope or answer for your child's illness.

However, it is almost never that simple. Most common colds and viruses these days can turn into something worse quickly. There are so many more viruses and bacterial infections in this day and age (than just a few years ago) that it makes diagnosis very hard for a doctor. Mostly, the doctors rely on your vital information and your recorded data to assess your child's sickness. Quite frankly, there are many times that the doctor simply cannot give your child medication because the cold or virus will not be affected by the antibiotics. Administering antibiotics unnecessarily can cause possible future immunity problems to your child. So chill out, be vigilant and understand that your doctor is not Super Man. He is just simply a man (or woman) trying to do the best for your sick baby.

Bottom line: You know your child is not behaving normal and you can't help him, only the doctor can! You are desperate for anything to help your child feel better, so when the doctor says, "Well, it's either a cold or a virus--- Call if his/her condition changes or becomes worse and be sure to administer plenty of fluids and allow the child to get lots of rest for the next few days." You then say,

"That's it? That's it? I paid a $20.00 co-pay for that?"

Yes, you did! Why? -Because you weren't monitoring and listening to your child as closely as you should be. *I am not trying to attack you as a parent or to say you have poor parenting skills.* Rather, we as parents need to tune into what our children are feeling. You should know by that mere change in their body functions when ailments are "just a cold/virus," or something much more serious.

I do not suggest that I always diagnose my children's sicknesses correctly. However, most of the time I have a pretty good idea of when they are sick, why they are sick, and what I can do about it (if anything). Here are a few tricks of the trade to help you beef up your skills to observe when your child is REALLY sick.

1. Think back to before they were sick (a few days before): Did you notice their urine smelling funny, off, or mediciny?

2. **How long have they had a fever?** If it is higher than 101°F, you need to be very vigilant. Someone once told me that if a child keeps a fever of 101°F or higher for more than 48 hours, it is bacterial. I do agree this seems to be the case more than not. Every time Julia has had a high fever and kept a fever, the cause has been (eventually) linked to a bacterial infection or childhood illness and not simply a "cold or virus."

3. **Is your child's nose stuffy, runny, does he have a cough or is he simply not breathing right?** There is a key difference. Having a cold is miserable enough, but when you can't breathe, you get the wheezing and the shallow panting, so watch for signs signaling your child could be in serious respiratory distress.

4. **Have they had very loose bowels?** This is another big sign that something is wrong. Too many stinky/nasty

diapers (with very foul odors) in a short period of time are a definite sign that something is wrong.

5. **Have they thrown up?** Projectile vomiting is different than food allergies or an "over-full" spit up. You will know the difference when it happens. Vomit from being to full kind of drips and dribbles down the mouth and front of the neck. Vomit that indicates your child is seriously ill will fly out of the mouth and your child will have no control over their body functions.

6. **Does your child's skin look rashy, blotchy, or crispy-white looking?** Rashes can indicate your child is sick, but more often than not, the sign of a rash comes toward the end of a sickness. A rash that appears like little red bumps right at the end of a cold, fever, or sickness, usually is the body's way of repairing the problem and getting rid of any residual ailment in your child's system. However, if you see a rash at the beginning of an illness, it could be a skin irritation of some sort requiring attention. Especially if the rash is accompanied by a high fever (Examples: hand, foot and mouth disease or the chicken pox). A rash can also be a sign of an allergic reaction such as a change in laundry detergent, a Christmas tree entering the house during the holidays, or a citrus or apple juice drink introduced recently to your child. A rash that accompanies 'Fifth's Disease or Slapped Cheek Disease' appears after the viral incubation period and there is nothing that can remove the rash other than time to get over the rash (which can be 3-40 days). I recommend reviewing the CDC (Centers for Disease Control and Prevention) website at www.cdc.gov to check out all the different symptoms associated with

different rashes. Also, check out this link at www.pediatrics.about.com/od/pictures to see pictures of many childhood diseases to help you identify what disease your child may have, if any (**WARNING:** Some images are graphic and disturbing!).

When you don't know, it can be scary!

It is so difficult to know when to take your child to the doctor. When Julia was in daycare, we took her to the doctor about twice a month with various colds, coughs and viruses. As time passed, we began to realize that our knowledge of when Julia was **really** sick was pretty good. In general, you will never miss the unmistakable white face that comes with red rosy cheeks and a listless behavior. This is usually always accompanied by a fever and your child will just fall into your arms for comfort. Vomiting and other signs, such as a rash, can also be symptoms of sickness. Most likely though, your child has a cold or virus passed around at school or nursery, and he or she will have to feel bad for a couple of days while the "creeping crud" passes.

Doctors have the tough task of telling you that you came to the office for nothing and to go home and give your child rest. I feel so sorry for patients and doctors because the patient only wants help and the doctor would love to help, but often can't intervene with Mother Nature's course of time that it takes to heal a cold or virus.

Having said that, don't just keep your children at home for extended periods of time when you know that something is "off." *Julia got croup once from daycare and by the third day, she was getting laryngitis (the adult form of croup). I was unaware of her serious symptoms because I didn't hear the "coughing seal" sound that everyone describes. Rather, Julia was just rasp, hoarse, and very tired. She wasn't really having trouble breathing until night time rolled around. When she would cry, I especially noticed a mousey squeak sound at the end of the cry that let me know she couldn't breathe well. I could tell she was beginning to take a turn for the worse the last evening before we showed up at the doctor's office.* As a parent, your parental instinct will play a key role in your child's health.

It will never hurt your child to go to the doctor and be sent home with no medications, however, you must expect this to happen every once in a while as there is nothing a doctor can do for a regular cold and cough. Some cough medicines and nasal decongestants can be prescribed, but over the counter medicine is so advanced these days that it is just as good as something prescribed unless the prescription has codeine in it to help your child rest and suppress their cough.

TRY THESE OVER THE COUNTER BUYS:	
Delsym (by UCB, Inc.)	for cough, up to 12 hours relief
Children's Benadryl® Allergy (by Pfizer)-	relieves allergy symptoms
Similasan	earache and pink eye, many more products as well
Little Noses products	decongestant drops and saline drops for cold and congestion

Trust your instincts:

Parenting is a life long journey, and the longer you are a parent, the more you will learn to trust your instincts. If you feel a little doubt or twinge that something is "off" then you need to go with it and see the doctor. Even if you are wrong, at least your kids are still okay and you don't miss the opportunity to help them feel better if they really are sick. I know beyond a shadow of a doubt that every parent can be in tune with their child. Just step back and watch their body language, their attitude, and their responsiveness (are they just whiny, sleepy, or are they really sick?). You have the innate ability to detect even the most minor ailments because you are their Mommy!

Colic tip:

I have a friend who said that catnip and fennel were good alternatives for treating colic. You can buy a mixture of these two herbs in herb stores in liquid drop formula. You need to speak with your pharmacist or herb care technician about how much to administer for your baby's weight, age, etc. However, my friend said that a maximum of ten drops was administered to her child's bottle each time and it seemed to help with the colic symptoms. Later, she decided to use the catnip/fennel formula every other bottle until she weaned her child from it completely.

My mother says giving a baby calcium-magnesium liquid will also help to ease colic. Tea tree oil is another alternative medicine that some people use for colic and one you should research thoroughly to see if it would be the best fit for helping your baby. Last, some mention sweet tea as a good remedy for treating colic.

WEANING is key:

Never stop taking a prescribed medicine cold turkey. A child must be weaned from any medications he or she may be taking for non-traditional purposes. Be sure if a medicine is not prescribed, that it is safe and in the correct dose for the child. Make sure it is in fact necessary. There are a lot of medicines available over the counter now, that we as parents have access to. You may think you are doing a good thing by giving your child fluoride, but if it isn't necessary don't give it to them (fluoride is provided in the city water systems). Always be sure to talk with your child's pediatrician before taking medicine rituals into your own hands. Remember, each of your children will be different with different needs to be met.

Medications:

Prescription medications are a wonderful life saver when you have been struggling with your child's illness. Be certain that the medicine prescribed is doing its job. If you have to wait a few days for the medicine to kick in, the doctor should tell you so. If you find that the medicine isn't helping, or worse, the medicine is making your child vomit, have diarrhea, have frequency of urination or cause them to be unbearably temperamental, be sure to call the doctor and ask to change medications and give the reasons and symptoms as to why this is necessary for your child. Investigate and remember to read the fine print on the medications prescribed. *Check the side effects of a drug; does it cause an increased frequency in urination?* If your child is experiencing a drug-related side effect that is bothersome, then by all means ask to change prescriptions for him or her. You are the adult. Doctors like a parent who can take control. If they don't, at least they know that when they deal with you, they must take you seriously.

CHAPTER 10
Don't forget about YOU!

Okay, it goes without saying that you are obviously in a marital relationship. If you are pregnant and with child, the next nine or ten months of your life will be totally consumed with the changes of your body and your mind. And then…when baby arrives you will experience even more changes and more "sacrifices" to meet everyone else's needs. -Particularly, the needs of your new little one.

Though these feelings and changes that are happening in your life are in fact the most important changes in your life, you must remember one key piece of advice: NEVER LET GO OF WHO YOU ARE! *Why do I think that this would happen to any of us?* As relationships change and grow, we all change to make relationships with others work. So, it is no surprise then, that you will be making a ton of changes in the next few years to accommodate your new family life. I have spoken with many women on this topic, some younger, but mostly older. Each of those women had the same underlying story: They tried to change to be the best mom/wife/girlfriend/friend they could be to someone because that someone wanted them to change. In looking back, the new persona they created was not the personality that their spouse fell in love with, hence the spouse/significant other fell out of love because of those changes. If you can relate to these words, stop your behavior right now and remember who you were right in the very beginning of your relationship. Rediscover the old YOU!

Although we are all subject to small changes, we should never change our "core" personality. You need to remain true to yourself first, or else you can never be true to your children and husband. Don't let life's demands or your husband's or children's demands consume your personality.

Often times, we women sacrifice to the "n^{th}" degree to make sure that everyone else is well taken care all the while we are falling apart at the seams. We are packing on pounds, letting our hair and makeup go, working all the time even after we step back in the door of our households. So, I am asking you today to do something very simple, get back in touch with yourself.

Now, as a new parent, I should hope that you haven't lost the "U" in you yet. But often times by this time in a marital relationship, you have already compromised and sacrificed enough to lose those little pieces of yourself in the mix. **Compromise is a good thing**, but only when it is done equally, so be sure that you are not always the giver and rarely the receiver. You need to hold your ground on important issues you believe in with all your heart! I think this is why women are so often called nags. By nature, women tend to agree with others and try to keep the peace. Finally, when the wife wants something or has a good idea, she has to nag the husband to death in order to finally "have a go" with that idea.

Why, in a book about children, do I include this topic? We as mothers give of ourselves so selflessly and without thought. We do what is inherent to nature, we give! Now, I am asking you to do what is not so easy, and that is "take" what you need to preserve your heart's happiness at this very moment. You need to remain "whole" inside to be the best mother you can be. If you let others chip away at your core being, you will only be a fraction of the "whole picture" that your child, 'soon to be,' will need for the rest of their life. So make a change now if this chapter applies to you. Regain your spirit and fight for what matters to you.

How do I take back my life?

I'm not going to talk about manicures, pedicures and the bubble bath you need to relax and reset your frame of mind. We've heard that enough to know that, "Yes, that would be nice, if I had the time." We've tried countless times to "make the time" to do these pleasurable things, but we are too busy in the mix of life to barely keep our toenails trimmed and painted. Much less treat ourselves with a soak in a soothing hot tub for an hour without our kids! Yum! That sounds great!

Instead of pampering yourself with undone relaxation techniques, I want to talk to you about getting back your core personality. The rules are simple and there is only one: **DO WHAT YOU NEED TO DO TO MAKE YOURSELF A HAPPY SOUL.** Now, I am not saying that you should just haphazardly go out and do whatever you want on a whim and not expect to have ramifications later. Rather, I am saying that you need to take a good look at the you that you used to like and then the you that you have become, and make key changes to rediscover that person inside you.

For the first 4 years of my marriage to Kurk, I tried so hard to please him and forgot completely about pleasing myself. In the course of all this "trying," neither of us really liked the person I became (though I felt he was changing me into this new 'person' while he felt I was becoming this 'person' on my own). Bottom line is that I forgot the essential me that I love, the me that I respect, and the me that I care about. When I decided I didn't like that "me" anymore, we had some huge marital issues associated with my will for a new lease on life.

Recently, I have been rediscovering myself, and it has been a long and slow journey toward a person I am beginning to like more and more. I find that this is not at all an easy journey, because once someone gets used to your being "stuck in a rut" they get rather used to your being in that "rut."

It takes some maneuvering, but it is possible to rediscover your old self and still be in your new life. I have learned that in order to be pleasing to everyone around me, I first have to please myself. I'm not talking about being greedy and taking everything materialistic for myself first. I'm talking about the principles of who you are and what you believe in. The "oomph" that made that person fall in love with you in the first place. Was it your outgoing spirit? Was it your ability to hold a conversation? Was it your funny jokes? You get the point.

Often, we forget to stay in tune with one another as spouses. We let so much of our relationship, and ourselves go. So work on getting back into shape, physically and mentally so that you can represent your family in a way that is positive not only for them, but mostly for you! Besides….you deserve the best YOU that you can be!

CHAPTER 11
Can this Marriage Survive?

I have come to the very real conclusion in life that each of our marriages is what we make them. You have the power to choose to invest your time and energy toward a positive relationship called "marriage" or face an eventual negative outcome we refer to as "divorce." You have to continually feed the "fire" you want to grow in a relationship. You also have to sacrifice or be able to 'meet in the middle' in a successful relationship. Ask of yourself no less than you would ask of your insurance agent who insures your home! Be sure you are investing your time and care in your marriage. It can be both as fragile as glass and as strong as steel.

I would be lying if I said Kurk and I had an easy time in our marriage. The truth is that some of it was rather tough. I want to make sure that you realize you are not the only one going through changes that happen in your married lives with children.

We are all going through life changes at different times because we are in different marriages. That does not mean you have to go through these changes alone. We should learn to talk more to each other. Sometimes, just talking to an understanding friend about your spouse can help alleviate the pressure so that you can 'de-stress' before trying to work things out with your spouse again.

I think so many of us are embarrassed to admit that our marriages have problems. However, sooner or later everyone will eventually know if you don't talk about your problems now. Choose a few points or main problems and start talking things out and getting them off your chest.

I want to deviate a little from my original purpose of this chapter and make a few general statements about trends or problems that occur in marriages. Rather, the outer lying circumstances we bring into our marriages which cause problems between two spouses.

I have compiled a list below of a few of the top sources of problems in most marriages with and without children. Some solutions are suggested for "meeting in the middle" **as a couple** to overcome differences and stresses in a marital relationship.

#1 problem in a marriage: MONEY PROBLEMS:

We all know the "no brainer" statement here that money continues to be the number one issue that most couples fight about, get divorced over, and ultimately, have to work for to support our broken families for most of our lives.

The love of money is a sneaky, evil, deep rooted ailment in American society. We all fall prey to wanting more of it, being concerned about when we aren't getting more of it, and making sure that we have enough of it to live our daily lives at the level we choose to live them. More specifically, a lack of enough money to support our ever lavish American life styles causes HUGE problems between spouses.

In a lot of marriages there is the "spender" and the "hoarder." One person might decide taking a quick weekend trip to the beach would be fun, never mind that you might drop an easy $500.00 in to a two-day fun filled excursion. The other might be considering how much money they want to put back on their 401K next year for their retirement savings. These are extreme examples, but my point is clear: **We don't always have the same idea as our spouse on how our money should be spent.** When you combine doctor bills, grocery bills, prescriptions, house payments, and utilities, the outlook becomes pretty dismal for the average American family. Even a family making a very nice $60,000.00 cannot really get much headway in this day and age without spending their money very carefully.

I think it should be very easy to agree that the income a family brings in becomes a key issue as to how it is spent as a family. I am a mother, and by nature have a huge instinct to want to go out and buy the cutest outfits, baby shoes and all the newest diapers, bottles and sippy cups. My ex-husband on the other hand, thought we had tons of sippy cups, "How could we possibly need more?" One might think that an extra $5.00 sippy cup on a bill would be a silly thing to argue about. However, when a wife comes home from the grocery store and the bill is twice what the husband expected it to be (God love the super stores these days) then you can't help but argue about how much money is spent at the store every week on a simple item like a sippy cup.

Kurk and I had discussed splitting our money up on several occasions, but truthfully it irritated me for him to suggest we have separate accounts.

I have a lot of friends that are remarried and feel that having separate accounts is the way to go in second marriages due to their separate children's expenses. However, when establishing a first marriage with children, I really think it is damaging to have two checking accounts. This scenario makes one person feel helpless (money deprived) while the other may have lots of extra income they could share with the lower paid spouse. I think for this reason alone, separate checking accounts can hurt self-esteem and create resentment between two people. By nature, people are very greedy and selfish about their money. Ultimately, money is what we work for day-in, day-out. We have to change our selfish, self serving ways and remember that if you are in a team, a team puts all their "rocks in a pile" and then distributes them among the wall to make a solid foundation. You cannot divide material wealth apart from one another and expect each person to feel equal in a marriage.

For me, it never mattered that I made less money than Kurk. However, I was always resentful when he suggested splitting up the banking account because I knew that gave me less spending money than him, and then I would feel indebted to him for any "extra" funds I spent on our family.

Budgeting is difficult!

I make a budget sheet every month like clock work, but where does it all go?

You can always count on an extra $200.00 being sucked right out the window before you even start to think of "extra money" at the end of every month. Quit making yourself miserable by not having extra money at the end of every month. Instead, try realizing that the cost of living with kids is expensive. And….. start enjoying your time with your family and realize in a few years after they get through all the viruses, colds and ailments passed on through the school system, your pocket book may finally feel some relief.

Start putting money back at tax return time!

It is really hard to save up and not spend the money that is 'in your face' every April at tax return time. If we would all learn to take our tax return and put away $1,500.00 or more immediately, then we would have that emergency money for the next year when car insurance, out-of-pocket health insurance or co-pays, and other unexpected expenditures pop up. You could even put all of your tax return in savings and have enough money for car repairs, vacations and Christmas presents at the end of the year if you could keep your sticky fingers from dipping into the kitty during the year. If you have money left over in January, consider taking that nice vacation in the spring with the extra funds.

Stop taking responsibility for family financial stress!

There is always one person in a relationship responsible for the bills. If the wife handles the checkbook and the husband is unhappy with the lack of money in the check book at the end of the month, sometimes the checkbook handler feels responsible. It is a hard thing to do but you must then hand over checkbook duty to the other spouse. Let the other spouse see how difficult it is to budget the funds with a family of four. Bills coming due at the 1st and

15th of the month can really make you feel broke one week, and rich the next week when you are paid. Juggling when to pay each bill, how to lump extra money together to do something useful with that money, and where to find the best bargain at the store to save money all become key factors when balancing the checkbook each month.

Fun money:

Agree to a certain amount each week of "fun" money for you and your spouse ($20.00 each is a good amount). Your fun money is also your "eating out money," your "let's go have a beer," money or your "let's go to the movies" money. Don't question your spouse about where their fun money goes during the week. Questions of accountability take the FUN out of fun money. Let them spend it however they choose (sometimes I buy Julia a gift or go out to eat with co-workers). If at the end of the week either you or your spouse have fun money left over, pool the remaining money together and split it equally between the two of you including your new fun money for the next week or take less fun money the next week and save money together. In this way, you are working as a team and you both experience give and take (one week you may have money left and your spouse may have none). Make sure you don't dip in to the checking account for extra "FUN" money during a week unless you both agree on it and can afford it in your budget.

Stop charging, start clearing!

Credit cards are a huge, huge problem for our generation. Did you know most of us carry $8,000.00 on average on a credit card? Stop! Plain and simple, just stop buying on credit. Stop buying all the things you don't need, and start putting away extra to pay off your credit cards. The payments suck up so much extra income. Also, it is not easy to recover financial stability once you get deep into unsecured credit card debt. Cut the card up, close the account if you have to (you can close an account and still pay on the balance with the account closed), but stop charging! Leave your credit card at home and make a deal with your spouse that you have to both agree to use the card before either one of you does the easy "swipe" on a machine. This way, you are serving as a final check for your spouse by asking "Do I really need this item or can I really justify a need for this item?" Bottom line folks: We are accountable to each other for our actions whether we like it or not.

Work together:

Money can divide and conquer your marriage! Don't give money the opportunity to drive a wedge between you and your spouse. Talk about your financial dreams, your financial goals and your financial needs before your next big purchase in your marriage. If the little purchases mean a lot to you or having lots of extra fun money is important to you, make that statement known in the beginning so that your spouse is clear on what your idea of financial happiness is when you begin to have a family of three, four or more! Remember to give a little on both ends: If you are the spender, learn to save a little and if you are the hoarder, learn to give a little. You will both ease up and depend on each other more to solve financial problems if you can realize that your spouse is your teammate and the best ally you can have in financial struggles of life.

#2 problem in a marriage:
THE EXTENDED FAMILY

Here we are; the number two topic of most married couple's woes, the extended family. How come when a couple first starts dating, the family seems to be sought after for approval and acceptance of a newly admired love? Once married, however, the couple pulls away from the family network. As their personal relationship develops, grudges are formed between the extended family and your personal relationship with your spouse. Before you know it, the spouse won't want to spend any time with extended family, they'll want their "personal goings on" kept private from extended family and last but not least, they'll want the family help only when they want it at their convenience.

Family is a VERY HARD topic to cover in this book because most of us either 1) love their family to the core and want to spend every waking moment with them; or 2) don't really care much about family and dread the holidays that force them to spend time with their extended family. Have you ever noticed with family there isn't really a person who is just "mediocre" with their family, they don't really care one way or the other? Many people grow up with strong roots to their family, holding that family relationship above and beyond everything else in life, even before their own marriages! Some people grow up wanting nothing more than to escape their families due to bad family history or circumstance. So what happens when you marry a person, live with them for years and learn that you both have a different idea of how involved your extended family should or shouldn't be in your life? Well, here within lies the reason for writing this chapter.

My family is very important to me, for years I put them first before absolutely anything in my life. Trying to please my father was my main goal up until age 27 or so.

So often, your family will become a "war zone" in your marriage. Your spouse may not like your parents, your brother or sister, the way you relate with someone in your family or a certain family member's ability to sway your opinions or outlook toward life and/or your marriage. In order to survive family, we must first understand where you fit into the puzzle we call "family."

Think back in to your childhood. What made you 'tick' as a child? What kind of child were you (happy, sad, lonely, or talkative)? It is the basis of your roots that you have grown and sewn which now make you the adult you are today. So, when you think of yourself now as an adult, a parent to a child yourself, ask yourself this question: "How can I make a difference in my family so that my children grow up realizing family is at the core of what is good about this world?"

I think greed, financial gain and hopes of success make each of us competitive in this day and age. We forget that we have a family who should be treated as such, and not a close knit group of people with whom we are competing. A common theme in every family is, "Who is doing what, who is earning what and who is saying what?" No matter what you think of each of your family members, you have to remember that you are not required to love them all the same, you are just required to love them all. Yes, you are!

--and if you can't give that love, at least treat them with respect!

Marrying someone who thinks and feels exactly about family as you do would be ideal. More often than not, we get crossed up in the misconception of family life and how exactly that relates to our personal relationship with our children and our spouse. So, here are some tips in relation to parenting and living with our extended family participating in our lives that might help you realize your way to a better familial relationship with your spouse and your extended family:

NEVER SECOND GUESS YOUR SPOUSE'S RELATIONSHIP WITH THEIR FAMILY

You may have a particular idea about how you have related with your family and how others should relate with their families. I can speak from my own personal experiences when I say that you need to let your spouse deal with their family the best way they know how. Often times, we as spouses want to jump in and assist, or change a bad relationship that may exist in your spouse's family. This is NOT a good idea as much as it may be at the heart of what seems good. Involving yourself to "fix" a familial problem between a sibling, parent or relative of your spouse will do nothing but come back to haunt you in future years. Resentment, anger and brute force for change will be felt by your spouse. Frankly, your spouse may be happy with the way things are whether you are happy with his/her familial relationships or not. Keep in mind that you should make sure your spouse has given every effort to make a relationship "good or right" with family members. If there is a reason for a hardship between two individuals, your spouse should state that reason to you so that you understand why they feel that way, and thus are able to accept the malfunction of that relationship. Often times, some relationships in a family are so damaged, that no attempt at repair can fix the broken bonds, and therefore, supporting your spouse's feelings on this broken relationship may ultimately bring you closer to your spouse.

It's human nature, we can't hold water

There are some things in life which you know you should not repeat to your spouse. However, it is human nature to want to say those unrepeatable phrases to your spouse to talk about how to fix them or get validations on a topic you may have spoken to a family member about. In passing on this conversation to your spouse, you could further create a barrier between you, your spouse and the clarity on which side of the line you stand on: Your family's side or your spouse's side.

Why does their have to be a side?

In general there is some discourse in most families, so naturally, yes; unfortunately there is a side to everything. Bottom line: learn to **not seek** validation from your spouse about things said with family members when you know in your heart it will only hurt your relationship with your spouse and your extended family.

Support your spouse unconditionally

This remains one of the very most important facts that I can relate to you about your relationship with your spouse and your family. I have found time after time a parent may not think that your spouse is honorable, or acceptable to their family circle. Instead of standing up for their spouses, husband and wives let their parents or relatives talk about their spouses negatively. This only creates a grudge if you relay information to your spouse about any judge of their character. The truth is that regardless of your family members statement's being valid or not, it is not their judgment call to make those statements to you or anyone else in your family. Furthermore, it is important for you as a spouse to let your family member know that you support your spouse, regardless of their mistakes, and that you do not appreciate them dividing you or putting a wedge between you and your spouse despite any personal indifferences within your marriage. It is not your family's job to point out wrong doings of your spouse; it is your job to notice them!

Talk to a family member that doesn't hold a grudge

So often we find a need to confide in our families about why our spouse may have upset us. Might I say that truly, it is nice to have a listening ear within your family circle, but rarely will you find a family member that can listen to your upset tone and then later not hold a grudge or "stack another brick" on the wall of honorability of your spouse. Therefore, you should confide in your family members with caution. However, finding a family member who is truly supportive and unbiased can be a huge help in wading through angry feelings in a relationship. Remember, anger can be worked out and fixed, but if your relative continues to be angry when you've long forgotten the reasons for your anger; then use caution when confiding in such an individual.

Agree not to let family persuade your attitude and ideas about life, in your marriage

So often we use our families as a sounding board for support and love when we have problems with our spouse. While support from family is good, sometimes it can be the 'finishing factor' on your marriage. If for example, a wife has always gone to her father for advice as a child, then the husband may feel that his personal ideas will always fall on deaf ears as he knows you will listen to your father instead. Likewise, a mother who is manipulative can manipulate her son and his marriage by imposing her ideas and beliefs on his marriage creating this stigma for a negative conduit between a husband and wife.

Please don't let your extended family persuade your ideas about your marriage. While taking advice to heart and applying some of those ideas to your marriage may be a good plan, we still need to remember to consider that our spouse also has a voice to be heard. Let's not forget that your spouse is the "other half" of your life, so make sure that when you open your ears to listen, you are listening to your married partner and not a family member in your extended family.

Establish rules for family visits

Whether you live a mile from your parents or you live 2,000 miles away, you must establish rules for family visits. Holidays especially seem to be the most stressful times for most of us as we try to visit everyone in our extended family over just a few days of the year. Remember, your spouse may not particularly enjoy your Uncle Ned, but will visit him twice a year because you like his family.

I used to think the idea of going to visit your family without your spouse was a crazy idea. However, sometimes your spouse may feel awkward or feel as though he doesn't fit in. If this situation happens, you may be missing out on quality family time trying to make your spouse feel a part of the situation when quite frankly, they'd rather be home. It is in this situation that going without the spouse may help alleviate pressure from both sides. Allow your spouse the freedom to choose not to come or participate with you, and then really take advantage of that time apart. He can work on things at home, while you spend much needed time with your parents and siblings catching up. The key factor is that if you both agree to spend time apart, then you should also both agree not to hold a grudge for one family member having spent that time with the extended family.

Don't ask for family help and then get mad when they don't do it your way

I think we all are guilty of asking our families for help and then realizing afterward that we should have just found a way to do it ourselves. I don't mean to say that asking for help from our own flesh and blood isn't a good idea. Rather, I think when we ask for our family's help, what we are really asking is for them to help us on our own terms.

More and more I see young Americans asking their parents to keep their children for them during the day as a solution to public daycare. Remember though, grandparents have the right to be grandparents. So, when you ask a grandparent to be an enforcer of rules and regulations toward their grandbaby, you have to realize the grandparent is going to treat their grandchildren the way they wish. In affect, you are asking your parent to "save you a buck" by watching your child and then getting mad when they don't watch them the way you want them too. *I ask you, what do you expect a grandparent to do?* It is a hard predicament for all parties involved. If however, you pay your parent to keep your child, a new set of rules apply because now you expect them to discipline your children on your terms as they are being paid to follow your instruction, in which I agree! Sadly, you must come to terms with the fact that your parents will never "lay down the law" and enforce the kind of parenting on your child that only a mother or father can enforce. Remember to be realistic of your expectations of your parent who truly wants to enjoy their grandchildren, and not go through a second lifetime of raising children.

Be sure when you involve another family member for help that you realize their form of help may not be what you visualize. To make sure that their help is actually helping, clear agendas and rules should be established before engaging in helping one another inside the confines of family. All involved must be open to communication including disagreements on the way their "help" is or is not working out.

Learn to enjoy your family again

What happened to the good ole' apple pie eating, baseball playing, good summer time family fun that used to be a big part of American life.

I myself must admit, I really dread a family reunion from time to time and I love family! So, why is it that we so desire to separate ourselves from our extended family in this day and age?

I think the main reason is that most of us don't have any "down time" to enjoy by ourselves. Therefore, we become super selfish with the time we do have to spend with our children and spouses, which doesn't amount to much.

We as a society should seek to change the direction we are moving our families in. Until we make a conscious effort to take the emphasis off money and material goods and start making choices for the good of our children, I'm not sure we can remedy the broken ties of family in this day and age. So, what I can say is you must do the best you can, try to focus on loving one another and really reaching out to each other with what little time you have. It is important for our children to know their cousins, their grandparents and their aunts and uncles; not as people they see a few times a year, but as real people who are involved in their lives so that those memories can translate into love which will last your child's lifetime.

#3 problem in a marriage:
SEX

Why cover the topic of sex in a book about life after birth? Truth is sex is either non-existent at this point or banging with exuberance (pardon the pun). Sex is such a weird and taboo topic, that I almost hesitate to cover it; yet, it is up there in the list of making a marriage "work" after having children. I only have a few things to say about sex because I do not in any way profess to be a "sexpert."

You must have meaningful sex in a relationship to remain together

Many men may not know this, but I think I can speak for a large majority of women out there when I say that most women could go their natural born life without having sex and still feel like life was worth living. Although sex is a beautiful and wonderful experience when you FINALLY figure out how to do it, sex has been correlated with so many bad experiences in an adult's life (i.e. broken hearts, affairs, etc.), that often we allow our minds to restrict us from enjoying it. Often, it's only the scandalous moments that allow one to enjoy sex when in reality you are probably tearing your life apart if you have reached that point. So, what I have to say about sex, attraction, marriage and life, although not ground breaking, may surprise even you.

Form a bond with your spouse like no other

It takes a pretty special man and woman who can argue one day and then make passionate love the next as if that argument never happened. Sex correlates to women as emotion, thoughts, and then actions. Sex correlates to men as actions, thoughts and then emotions. So, how in the world do a husband and wife meet in the middle in the same room, after years of marriage to still enjoy that intimate relationship without getting bored? Well, it's not easy. But, with a few tips, more emotional than sexual (we all can 'do it' by this age) maybe we can start to realize what makes the opposite sex tic so that we can enjoy sex without inhibitions.

First, trust is key

So often, jealousy, lack of trust and feelings of ownership tear down the pure beauty of a sexual relationship. It's hard to understand why some people have jealousy in their heart and an unwillingness to trust a spouse, yet those characteristics are a part of their life based on past personal experiences. *I have often said to my girlfriends, "What I don't know won't hurt me." A lot of that holds true. I have spent many relationships trying to sneak around and "catch my partner" in the act of doing something wrong. Why? I'm only hurting myself here. And, if I got caught trying to catch them 'in the act' it only proved worse for ware on the relationship.* I do really feel that you should trust that your partner is being faithful until you have reason to doubt. Always doubting, feeling that weakness in your mind and heart, never, ever translates to beautiful love between two people. The way I see it, you have to trust from the very beginning that someone will be faithful, until they give you a reason not to trust them. You should not harbor jealousy, anger or doubt.

---And honestly, do you really want to be with someone if you can't trust them or if you have to watch them 24/7 to keep them from cheating on you? Really, you are bigger than that, so your answer here should be, "No."

If you sense a cheating heart, you are probably not far from wrong

I'm definitely NOT talking about searching out someone's infidelity. I'm not talking about checking up on someone to catch them in a lie. What I'm talking about here is the 'err' of someone's demeanor which makes you feel uncomfortable when that individual is around your spouse. *Have you ever disliked a co-worker of your spouse or felt like that co-worker had feelings for your spouse? Have you ever approached your spouse about a co-worker or friend who you felt might be sending the wrong messages and your spouse flatly denied that those feelings may be being projected towards them?*

I think talking about an attraction that someone may have toward your spouse is a healthy start. Even if your spouse disagrees with your point of view on an individual's actions, making the point in itself will cause your spouse to be wary of that individual if your spouse has an honest heart.

Let's face it though girls! All women are attractive, especially after you get to know them. I find so many people intriguing and charismatic; their exuberant personalities seem to highlight their feminine qualities even more. So, you can see how in a weak moment, (which we all have as human beings) huge mistakes can be made. Therefore, it is very important for you to realize that **your husband (or wife) is obtainable to someone else, no matter how happy your marriage may be**. You have got to walk a fine line against that fictitious individual out there always threatening to take your LIFE away. Now, am I saying you should be doubtful of everyone, close minded and down right jealous? No. I'm saying the opportunity exists at any given time on any given day, to make a mistake as a spouse.

<u>Bottom line:</u> You have to protect your marriage, make your marriage strong, and point out those weaknesses to each other. -Bind together to hold the course so that nothing will be able to steer your family in the wrong direction.

For example, if you invite a wayward person into your home because you may feel sorry for them, then don't wonder why your spouse ends up cheating with them. This person who is alone may need that "rush" to feel alive again. Your spouse could be the answer to their void in their personal life. You cannot create an opportunity for misfortune; rather, create a strong bond as a couple to safeguard your relationship from these types of circumstances.

#4 problem in a marriage:
Life Stress:

Have you ever been so busy being angry about a situation involving work or home that you can't enjoy the limited time you have with your spouse or your children?

Why do individuals make other people's problems their own?

By human nature, I think a lot of us desire to cause strife in our own lives. It's like a gushy novel come to life for each of us to sort out in living color! Otherwise, we would be bored or happy which are the alternatives to strife. So, since being happy 24/7 is not possible for most people, we choose to talk about others and bring other people's problems into our own lives so that we can "fix" everything for everyone around us, except for ourselves!!!! Big NEWS FLASH folks: AN OLD DOG CAN'T LEARN NEW TRICKS. Nor can you pressure, push or threaten anyone into changing their life/lives without their willingness to change. Believe me, I have tried COUNTLESS times to yell, scream and beat the truth (or my version of what I believed to be the truth) into someone's head in order to better themselves. Quite frankly, most people are addicted to the financial stress, a bad situation, or an attitude they present to the world…because if they wanted too…they could change these weak points in their lives starting today!

Instead of trying to fix the world as you've been doing for so many years, might I suggest you try and fix yourself first?

Focus on taking responsibility for your own actions, for your own attitude and the way you project yourself to others on a daily basis. Do you walk into a room and smile or do you cringe and grumble? Do you find time to ask someone how they are doing or do you immediately talk about yourself the whole time you spend with a friend? Marriage, love, friendship and children all require willingness to give and take on a continual basis.

How much of yourself do you give?

If you give too much, start taking some of life for yourself.

How much do you take of/from others?

If your answer is too much and truly you know if you are one of these individuals, then start to give that time/energy in return to others.

It's really quite simple: Life is a two-way street and if you tear down one side of the road and never look to see who is coming down the opposite side of the road, nor what is on the side of the road in the tree line; eventually you will crash and burn due to your blind sighted attitude. Don't let this happen to you. Learn to destress, pay attention and focus on your own person. Then you will begin to realize that what is happening around you is part of life, and not necessarily your problem to pick apart and fix. Focus on yourself, your attitude and your ability to affect relationships around you. Honestly, life simply is a carnival ride, don't pick it apart; just enjoy it for what it is. Here are some ideas to destress, renew and start focusing on what's important.

Constructive destressing:

If you choose to confide in a friend about and argument with your spouse, be sure the friend is a forgiving friend. You do not want to tell your best friend about a heated argument between you and your spouse only to find out years later that she is holding a grudge against your husband for the way he treated you during a past incident. Friends should be supportive. Remember all people say things they shouldn't say and do things they shouldn't do in the heat of an argument. I'm not trying to justify any bad behavior, rather, I am trying to point out that what may seem cruel or malicious to you may not seem cruel or malicious to the next individual. Not everybody "fights fair" or at the same level you may (some people never fight, some people fight constantly, it's their way of life).

A listening ear:

As a friend, having a listening ear is the best support you can give a friend in need of advice. Your advice doesn't have to be direct nor does it have to be specific. Words of encouragement such as "I know you will figure out the best choice for you;" or "That sounds like a great idea to help work things out," can be simple statements of validation that your friend is searching for. Most friends just want confirmation that the feelings they have about a particular disagreement are valid feelings. A person wants to feel understood, if not by a spouse, then by a friend. That's why they turn to you. Getting angry along with your friend who is conveying an upsetting story to you is not necessarily an emotion your friend wants you to feel. Instead, try offering supportive words and help that individual pick a good scenario to solve their problem(s) with their spouse. Most of the time a person already has an idea of how to solve a disagreement; they just want your opinion on what might be the right direction to start the healing process.

A word on friendship:

I'll try not to open my mouth too wide here for fear that a foot might come flying right back at me. I have no doubt screwed up my share of friendships, but I have also learned a thing or two about how to cultivate and maintain a life long friend. Friendships are one of the main things in your lifetime that will keep you sane and resilient during some of the rockiest times of your life. Therefore, you have to know a thing or two about give and take, love and losing, sharing and hording, and mostly, showing up when it matters most.

There are defining moments in each friendship's cross roads when you ask yourself, is this friendship really worth keeping?

And though I think some of those moments that define them can be rather heart wrenching, I must say that every friendship, just as a marriage, is worth a fighting battle.

You must understand that each of us was raised in different backgrounds, different environments of learning, and different parental influences. That makes us, well, quite different! So, in order to cultivate a friendship with people who are much different than you (it can be done) you must see the world through their eyes. Try to be more flexible and sympathetic to others' needs and remember, even if those needs seem corny to you, they are important to your friend.

I have a girlfriend whose husband is a doctor. She is currently in graduate school and has little time to spend with her spouse. He is a pediatrician and is on call and working most days and their time together is very minimal. Therefore, if she cancels on me and our planned lunch at the last minute (and I always bring my lunch to work in case this happens) I don't have my feelings hurt at all. I realize that her relationship with her husband comes first, and I appreciate her dedication to spend as much time with him as possible.

You have got to stop taking things so personally in relationships and realize that everyone in life is not going about their day scheming to hurt you. Furthermore, did you ever think that maybe your friend is going through a hardship they haven't cared to share with you, and they need that special time with their spouse to make things right?

It seems the older we get as adults, the less open and sharing we become with our feelings and relationships. Some of that is okay, but other times it can be destructive hanging on to all the baggage ("Our own sack of rocks" as my Dad likes to call it).

Solving a problem could be quite different for you versus your friends' solution due to each of your personalities and personal experiences. For example, I might tell one friend how beautiful they are, but I may not say the same to another friend because they may be less comfortable with my describing them in such a way. Some girls are very "girly" and tend to be drama queens, while others are quiet and more reserved (more like a male counterpart when it comes to emotions). This doesn't mean you are less compatible as friends. If you are a drama queen and your friend is not, then use similarities and passion for life as the basis of maintaining that friendship.

#5 problem in a marriage
Letting yourself go:

Men want their wives to stay just the way they looked when they started dating and remain that way for the duration of their relationship. While women want their men to meet their emotional needs first and then the man's physical appearance becomes important after their emotional needs are met.

This is why a somewhat average looking male can be seen with a gorgeous female. He meets her emotional needs and his looks play second fiddle. It is no surprise that if you are a walking and talking female, you should know that the majority of men desire a woman who looks and feels her best! Stress of a full-time job and your focus on the children will no doubt allow your physical appearance to suffer. You must work hard to get yourself back in shape (not thin ladies, just shapely) and get your self-esteem rolling like a freight train. Even if you are not who you used to be, you can create a "new" and better you that you can be proud of and love just as much. Investigate what is on the inside to find the person you really want to become on the outside and go from there. Don't let others (your spouse included) beat you down about your looks; instead focus on where you want to be when you are healthy every day. And "just do it!"

So many husbands and wives have their version on what a healthy partner should be like. Maybe healthy to you means a "thin" appearance, while healthy to another individual means that they exercise every day regardless of their waste line size. *I think that the health of an individual must start in their mind and grow outward. If you do not have a positive attitude and a healthy outlook on life, then certainly you will never have a healthy body, regardless of your size or shape.*

I struggle EVERY DAY with my health. Some days I feel like working out and for the life of me, I cannot make the time in my schedule to do it. Truth is, when I really want to work out, I do. So, let's not forget that health first is a state of mind which translates into a physical action once we get our mind healthy.

Why won't the weight come off?

There are only three solutions to this question:
1) You're eating too much or your diet is poor
2) You're not exercising enough
3) You're genetically pre-disposed to weight gain

If any or all of the choices above apply to you, you've got to figure out what is most important to you and to your marriage. Will your spouse continue to love a heavier you? Will your spouse resent that you have "let yourself go" and seek alternative satisfaction outside your marriage? More importantly, will you love yourself as a heavier individual and will you feel comfortable in your new clothing size?

It is very hard for me to accept that I may never be a size 10 again. In fact, most of the time I wonder when and how I will lose weight because truly I feel in my heart I want to be thin. It is very difficult to find the time in my schedule to want to take time out for me. I'm so selfish to want to rush home to be with my kids that I forget in the long run it is me that gets neglected. How do I fix this pattern of self destruction?

We have to make the decision to get on an exercise program because most of us love to eat! I know very few women who "eat to live." Most women "live to eat." Therefore, if you choose to continue to consume the foods which we all desire most (high fat, low nutrition) then we've got to make a sacrifice somewhere along the way......

Shall I work out? Or shall I eat smaller portions of better foods?

I hope the answer is that you will make a conscious effort to both work out and eat less. Working out doesn't mean going to a gym and climbing on a treadmill every day, although admittedly, if you want to lose weight and keep it off, you have to learn to incorporate exercise into your daily routine. Working out can simply mean walking briskly for 30 minutes a day and lifting weights on alternate days. Try an elliptical machine with an easy stride and a low impact work out for starters to help you move toward a healthier you.

Weight loss drugs:

I'm pretty sure most of us in our late 20s to early 30s by now have tried every weight loss drug on the market, even those prescribed by your doctor. Dieting, pills, and starvation seem to be the only way for most of us to lose the extra weight. Hey, you may look good, but it makes for a cranky pilled up starving wife most of the time...... how's that for a happy marriage?

A lot of my friends, including myself, have reported very irritable behavior while on weight loss drugs. Not only do the prescribed drugs tend to keep you awake at night, they also make you cranky and irritable. Some of my friends have noticed considerable hair loss as well as fading in sexual desire while the appetite suppressing activity tends to "fade off" after just a few weeks on the drug.

However, weight loss drugs can be nice because they can help you get that new and exciting thinner look relatively quickly. But let's be frank here: How many of us work out long enough to keep all those lost pounds off?

Unless you work out and maintain smaller portions (hard to do once off the drug) then it is really hard to keep all those lost pounds off. I think in discussing a healthier "you" we should discuss a sensible "you" as well. If you realistically believe that you can continue to eat smaller portions and make healthier food choices once you are off of the weight loss drug <u>AND</u> you have considered all of the drug's side effects, then go for it. However, if realistically you know that you will not maintain a program adhering to healthier eating styles after you have taken the drug and lost the weight, then might I suggest that until you are ready to "go at it" full force, you put the physical part on the back burner and focus on your mental health instead. Mental health as I said before is the first step toward a healthier you, and there is no shame in starting small and taking "tiny bites" toward your long term goal.

I want to be thinner but honestly I don't want it enough to eat less because I love food. So for now, I focus on trying to eat better, and trying to eat less. Yes! I get frustrated with my weight, but I realize that soon I will have the mental strength to create a new healthier me and that is what I strive toward daily.

Once you have established good health mentally, the physical aspect of getting in shape basically boils down to the amount of time you have to commit to an exercise program. I strongly recommend the book "Body-for-LIFE" by Bill Phillips, or go to www.bodyforlife.com to get tips on how to create a better, healthier you (he's the physical expert, so I'll let him tell you how to work the pounds off the right way and keep them off).

TIP:

One thing that helped me when I finally started back at the gym 2.5 years later after having my first child was to focus on pants sizes versus how many pounds I lost. Clearly, I was too far away from my goal weight to get excited about losing 5 pounds. However, a girl in the gym that I know who had lost a ton of weight said she focused on her pants size instead of watching the numbers so much (although that doesn't mean you have to avoid weighing unless you are a fanatic and let the numbers get you down). So, I have tried focusing on envisioning myself in size 10's (I'm not there yet). Every day when I am on the track and finding an excuse not to jog, I realize if I ever want to fit in my size 10's, I've got to get moving. To date, I am wearing pants that I couldn't even fit over my hips 4 months ago. That's progress! Only 15 pounds, but still progress because I go in to my closet and I find a new (old) pair of jeans that fit again and it is such a proud moment for me each time this happens.

#6 problem in a marriage
A marriage in strife:

If your marriage is already beyond the point of 'repair' then I would like to suggest that you reach out for help. No, I'm not speaking of an intervention where a group of people get together to tell you that your marriage is in dire straights. I am talking about admitting to yourself and your spouse that it is time to get help for your marriage, and then act on the realization that without it, your marriage could be on the outs, for good!

It is hard to know what is right in any marriage and what makes each person get through the day at a happy go lucky pace. Some people tend to be very high strung and anything can "set them off." Others can have numerous things go wrong through out the day and chalk it up to "waking up on the wrong side of the bed," and they'll just start over tomorrow.

When you feel at wits end, when you feel like you are so close to walking out that door that the mere thought of the freedom from the "chains of your marriage" gives you relief to just think about it. ---Then you, my friend, are the one I am talking to.

Having said that, let me assure you that you will know when you need the help…and if you admit to yourself that you are having these feelings, then that is the biggest and first step in the right direction.

Might I suggest that this is the time you need to reach out the most?

Don't forget about your close non-judgmental friends. I assure you, if you will just talk to them you will find that some of them have been through it too (something about having a second child seems to bring on too much strain in the modern day family, and for some reason, this is usually the breaking point in most young marriages, and unfortunately, your children's young lives).

If you are a firm believer that medicine and counseling aren't necessary to help you through rocky times, then you may **miss the only "boat" to an easier ride through the rough, rocky waters in your marriage.** *Now, I am not suggesting you go get drugged up to numb yourself from the pain.* However, I am saying that most women have an array of emotions both during pregnancy and after pregnancy. These emotions may well up and explode like a demon with a death wish. It is an uncontrollable surge of sheer anger or contempt that digs down into the depths of your mental capacities and seethes out the edges of your eyes, and erupts from your mouth when you speak. If you think this is happening to you then you may need a mood altering drug. I am not suggesting that you take this drug for the rest of your life. Rather, I am suggesting for your sanity and ability to exist in your own body for a period of time, you should talk to your doctor about the possibility of some chemical assistance.

The following drugs are some of the most popular 'mood levelers' on the market today: Wellbutrin, Prozac, Zoloft, Paxil, and Effexor. Discuss your options with your doctor and don't be afraid to cover the topic of sexual inhibitors. Some of the anti-depressant/mood leveling drugs can have an effect on your desire to have sex. Before committing to a prescription drug, request samples from your doctor's office if available to be sure that you find the right mood leveler for your needs.

Another self-help topic is that of counseling which I feel is needed in every relationship. A relationship that is going quite well or one that is on the outs, still needs counseling to learn how to truly communicate with one another.

My ex-husband and I had been through our share of ups and downs. Something I found more annoying than anything was that even during our "up" times we were still holding on to grudges from the "down" times that bubbled up and exploded over during simple arguments. I don't understand why, but sometimes it is very difficult to communicate with a spouse.

To compound the marriage obstacles of verbal discussions, you have past perceptions of one another from past experiences. There is an old saying that "everyone has their own sack of rocks to carry….(baggage along the way)." Husbands and wives often may bring up these past occurrences during new confrontations further beating down each other's self assurance and esteem. I think that counseling is a good answer for everyone in marriage when they are having a difficult time communicating such as these experiences described above.

Let me state for the record that I don't know many men who believe in counseling, and a lot of women also think it is a joke due to the over-popularization of the TV image of a "shrink." If you will just go and give it a chance and open up your heart, and speak the truth and the reason you are sitting in their office from the onset and what you hope to accomplish from your meetings; I promise you that counseling will pay off.

---And, if your spouse won't attend, go by yourself. The anger and hurt in your heart that you can release is tremendous, and the ability to communicate, empathize, sympathize, strategies to disengage anger, and learn how to work together with your spouse;

will help you make counseling a tool for solutions to many marital problems.

CHAPTER 12
You can Make it!

I have to agree with Dr. Phil on this one (who I used to think was a quack, before I realized I was the quack and he was the one actually doing something about it) and say that you need to try try again, and explore every avenue to fix your marriage before you go through the damaging and final step of separation and divorce. We do give up way to easily as married couples in this day and age, and people who generally make great couples end up divorcing over issues that they can't seem to agree on. Furthermore, the work force and lack of togetherness of family can drive a wedge right down the center of your "family time" and cause you to avoid sitting at a table together and enjoying each other's company, or watching a movie or going to the park together. You need to ask yourself "Why am I in this marriage?" and if you can't find a good reason or answer to that question, you need to seek your spouse out and be sure you can say, "It is because I love you and I like it that we are a part of each other's life, you make my world whole and complete." So work on these skills of really talking it out, saying what you mean and not keeping your feelings bottled up inside. I promise your rewards will be so fulfilling, you will wonder how come you've let unspoken feelings go on this long. Be sure to talk things out and explain to your spouse what your life needs NOW that will make you want a long term commitment that can last your lifetime.

And from here, we live on!

I would like to close this book by saying that every day is a challenge and battle in your new life that you have begun with your family of three….and more. I want you to really connect with those around you, to reach out to your support network (and create one if you don't have one) and be secure in telling that one friend your deepest feelings so that you can get feedback on the fact that you aren't the only one to have felt "that" in the history of mankind. I want you to be more open, more flexible, and more forgiving of mistakes that we as family members and spouses make toward one another.

Don't forget, there are little ones watching your EVERY move and they are learning by example on a daily basis. In order to be the parent you want to be, you have to live the life that you know needs to be lived, correctly. That not only starts from the mental and physical points of view (being mentally capable, and physically in good shape to handle your daily routine) but also involves being generous, caring, reflective, understanding, and sometimes even selfish in some aspects of every day living. You have got to remember when to stand up and "fight the good fight" and then when to sit down and let the "waves roll on." I need you to be strong for you first, your spouse next, and your children after that. Incorporating God in your life can make a difference, and religion can help build that religious network that is so desperately missing from many family's homes in this day and age.

This book is not just about the "nows and what is happening today….," but it is also about the "where are we going from here and what do we want out of our lives?," that I am asking of you.

Your children should be the number one important topic in your everyday life, and you have to ask yourself how can you strive to make a difference, a measurable difference in their little worlds each day. To love a child is like loving your own self because you should do it completely and unconditionally, but with careful thought. If you can't love yourself first, then you should work on that, as your children will see this void in you.

Remember, life is good, and you make each day your own, so don't throw away your today and your tomorrows on wasted time, wasted words, wasted money and wasted attitude. Rather, set your sights high, and remember your children are counting on you!

EPILOGUE

As I write these words on paper, I wonder what my children are doing at home with their Nana. The precious moments that slip away daily are so very valuable, and only for a time. Yet, I am proud that my children have their grandmother there to nurture their little souls daily and that she takes care of my most precious treasures: my children!

Life is not perfect. Rather, life in fact is so much more than we bargain for sometimes. Each person has their own personality that adds to the mix we call "life." I am so proud of each parent who strives to be the best they can be for their children without trying to hold up to unrealistic expectations. We live each day, we love each day, and every day should be cherished as the last because we know not what the morrow may bring.

Communication with friends, family, doctors, and associates will prove most vital, and your most needed skill in order to make your life easier and more fulfilling. You have to learn to be a more understanding, well rounded individual. Have the ability to sit back and "watch life" without stressing out about every little detail. Remember to always show compassion, give of yourself what you expect of others and show everyone that your model would be the one to emulate.

Share your happiness, your secrets, your tips and your daily rituals with others. Don't be so closed minded and quick to the "exit ramp" when you could be helping someone else figure out something that you now know how to do with ease. Talking between friends sometimes opens doors that you never expected to fly open. Mostly, keeping abreast of the current events of your children's lives and sharing important tips you have discovered keeps the lines of communication open. Don't be afraid to ask how to clean that belly button lint out, or what your best friend did when she went into labor. Don't forget to ask about the simple things, like how much easier changing a diaper is if you put the other diaper underneath it first (Secret's of the Baby Whisperer tip). Mainly, just share your thoughts, but in a loving way and not a bossy way. Learning the art of speech is something each of us should strive to do every day. I still trip and stumble daily, but bottom line is: I TRY!!!!!

Children are the door way to our future, folks! They are the new leaders of tomorrow. They hold my dreams, my inspirations, my hopes and thoughts in each and every smile I see on their faces daily. Cherish your children and love them with a wholeness and completeness that at times you find it hard to muster up the energy within yourself. And remember, the love you give your children will reflect through their tiny little spirits and shine outward because your children are mirrors of what you teach them to be.

Last, love yourself first! Love yourself completely! Love the relationship you are in and find a way to rekindle that love if you have long since let that flame die out. Give yourself the ultimate care and the responsiveness that a parent seeking to help their newborn child would give. You are what you make, and from this day forward, you can choose to make yourself the person you want to be. Strive to be a person who will be more relaxed, less stressed, more truthful and gossip less about life. People are watching you to see how you raise your children. Let's show the world that whether or not you are a working parent in the work force, a working parent at home, or a mix of the two, that each one of us has something special to offer our children!

God Bless each of you, keep your heart healthy, your children safe, and your smile right side up!

Love
Britton

DAILY ACTIVITY SHEET

Name: _____ **Date:** _____

MORNING

BREAKFAST:

I had
- _____
- _____
- _____

And ate: LITTLE   SOME   LOTS

BOTTLES:
- _____ OZ TIME _____
- _____ OZ TIME _____
- _____ OZ TIME _____

DIAPERS:
- TIME _____ WET BM
- TIME _____ WET BM
- TIME _____ WET BM

Fever noticed, temp of: _____ °F at _____ AM/PM

NAP: _____ HRS

AFTERNOON

LUNCH:

I had
- _____
- _____
- _____

And ate: LITTLE   SOME   LOTS

BOTTLES:
- _____ OZ TIME _____
- _____ OZ TIME _____
- _____ OZ TIME _____

DIAPERS:
- TIME _____ WET BM
- TIME _____ WET BM
- TIME _____ WET BM

NAP: _____ HRS

GENERAL NOTES FOR PARENT OR DAYCARE:

(Example: Medicine to be given at certain times today or if child was sick today)

_____
_____

I NEED: DIAPERS   WIPES   FORMULA   BABY FOOD   JUICE

OTHER: _____

PARENT'S NUMBERS:

MOM, NAME:
Work:
Cell:
Other:
Emergency contact:

DAD, NAME:
Work
Cell:
Other:
Emergency contact:

Picture of your child here

INDEX

A

After child birth
bleeding 19-21
body reactions 18
eating 19
husband 28-30
ice pack 17
nurses helping 21-23
periods 46-47, 88-90
swelling 18

B

Baby acne 38
Baby rash: Desitin and
   Vaseline 32-34
using Clotrimazole 1%
   (Antifungal cream) 39
using Hydrocortisone 1% 39
Bathing and toweling 30-32
Bathroom: after birth 20-21
Birth control
and break through
   bleeding 47, 89-90
brands and mood issues 90
switching after pregnancy 89
while breast feeding 68
Body parts: Cleaning and….
belly button 37
ears, nose & toes 38

Body reactions after
   child birth 18
Bottles & Nipples:
specific bottles 86-88
sterilizing 85
using bleach 85-86
using dishwasher for 85
when to throw away 86
Breast milk:
how long is it good for 88
in freezer bags 88
mixing with formula 76
not producing enough 77-82
production of during a
   work week 76, 80
Breast Pump
brand to buy 74-75
used pumps 74
when to buy 75
Breastfeeding
and pamp smear results 42
at nurses stations 84-85
at work 83-85
before let down 78-79
choosing between breast
   or bottle 68-70
choosing to pump 69
how long does it take 72
in bed 81-82

positions for 81-82
stopping/weaning 82
with disgression 83-84
your rights 83-84
Breasts:
infections of 72
painful to touch, red
   and streaky, 72

C

Cancer 41-43
Car seat
putting car seat in car 25
Carcinogens 41
Cervix: size after birth 22
Cheating 138-139
Cholestoral 43-44
Circumcision tips for
   care 32-33
Colic
remedies to try 114

D

Daycare 56-59
in home daycare 59-60
mommy daycare 62-64
options: see work options
pros and cons 55-58
sick kids in 58
Diaper rash 36-37
Diapers 36
Diet pills 46, 147-148

Dieting 145-149
Doula 13

E

Exercising and goals 149

F

Family
definition of extended
   family 11
enjoying family
   again 135-136
family help 134-135
family persuasion 133
family visits 133-134
gossip among family 131
spousal support 131-132
talking with family 132
your spouse's family 130-131
Formula:
and mixing with
   breast milk 76
Nestle Good Start 76
Friendship 143-145

G

Good buy tips:
bed rails 93
eBay 93
Evenflo milk storage
   bottles 87
Nestle Good Start formula 76

Olan Mills 96-97
One Step Ahead
   magazine 91, 93
Playtex Nurser Bottles 88
Pump In Style Breast Pump
   by Medela, Inc. 74
Secrets of the Baby Whisperer
   (Tracy Hogg) 73
Good tips:
baby gates and door
   locks 99-100
book clubs 94
bras & tank tops 98
changing tables 92
cheap baby proofing 100
child waking in the night 99
colic tip 114
diaper scents/sense 92
discount stores 95
mom's wardrobe 104-105
parent pages on the web 101
passing down baby
   clothes 101-102
pictures of children 96-97
size doesn't matter 103-104
Watch Me Grow
   Picture Club 97

H

Hair loss 45-46
Help 151
Hemorrhoids

and processed foods 45
cream for 45
vitamin B6 for 45
Home
doing to much once
   home 27-30
the rest of your life 27
Hormone levels 18, 28
Hospital stay:
staying full length of
   time 22-23, 28
help from others 17-
   18, 21-22, 29-30
Hospital supplies
what to stock up on 23
Husband after child
   birth 28-30

I

Ice packs after child
   birth 17-18

J

Jealousy 138-139
Job options 52-53
Kegels
Kegels 16

L

Laxatives: for children 35
La Leche League
   International 83-84

Letting yourself go   145-149

M

Marriage and children 156
Extended family:
enjoying family again   135-136
family help   134-135
family persuasion   133
family visits   133-134
gossip among family   131
spousal support   131-132
talking with family   132
your spouse's family   130-131
Making a difference   156-157
Making it work   150-153
not giving up   155
Money problems   122-128
  credit cards   127
  family financial
    stress   125-126
  fun money   126
  saving money   125
Medications:
mood altering   151
prescribed and 'over-the-
    counter'   113, 151
side effects from   115-116
weaning from   115
Mental health   117-
    120, 148-149
Milk production:
breastfeeding for   67-70
drinking water for   78
herbs to avoid during   82-83
herbs to increase   82
less stress for   79
massaging your breasts for   79
slowly decreasing   80
taking Reglan for   77-79
when will it start after
    birth   71-73
Money
  credit cards   127
  family financial
    stress   125-126
  fun money   126
  saving money   125

N

Nipples and pacifiers
flow of nipple   87
how to choose brand   87
type of nipple   86-88
Nipples (breast):
cracking, scabbing,
    burning   73
relief with lanolin cream   73
Nurses helping after
    childbirth   21

O

P

Pacifiers

and boiling 86
Pain:
back and shoulders 23-24
relievers: Tylenol and Motrin 24
Pap smears 41-42
Parenthood 10-11
Periods
after pregnancy 46-47
and break through bleeding 47, 88-90
and frequency 88-90
and messed up cycle 88-90
while breast feeding 68
Pitocin 14
Pooping 14, 34-37
Pumping (See Breast Pump) 68
Pumping mother's rights 83
"PUSHING" during labor 15-16

Q

R

Reglan (for milk production) 77-79
Religion 156
Remember you 117-120

S

Sex: 136
cheating 138-139
meaningful sex 137
spousal bond 137
trust 138
Sick Child
and a doctor's point of view 108-109
colds & viruses 109
colic tip 114
fever 110
how to diagnose 110-112
loose bowels 110-111
signs of illness 110-112, 114
skin appearance 111
vomiting 111
when to take child to doctor 113
Skin problems (sensitive) 38
recipe for cream to apply 39
soaps for 38
Stress 140
constructive destressing 142
listening ears 142-143
Strife 150
counseling 151-153
medications 151
Supplies (needed from hospital or store) 23

T

Taking back your life 119
Thyroid problems 46

U

V

W

Websites recommended:
Bras & clothes: www.motherhood.com 98, 104
Centers for Disease Control: www.cdc.gov 111
Cholesterol: www.parentsplace.com/features/heart/qas/0,,239248_106143,00.html 44
E-Bay: www.ebay.com 93
Gerber baby food & charts for feeding: www.gerber.com/home 101
Herb-breast milk interactions chart: www.babycenter.com/general/8788.html. 82
La Leche League International: www.lalecheleague.org 83
One Step Ahead magazine: www.onestepahead.com 91, 93
Pampers for diapers and stages of baby growth: us.pampers.com/en_US/home/home.jsp 101
Pictures for pediatric illnesses: www.pediatrics.about.com/od/pictures 112
Tracy Hogg: www.babywhisperer.com/babywhisperer.html 73, 82
Weight loss drugs and behavior 147-148

Work options
back to work 52
from home 52
part time 52
shift scheduling 53
Working mom 49

X

Y

Yeast infections 37

Z

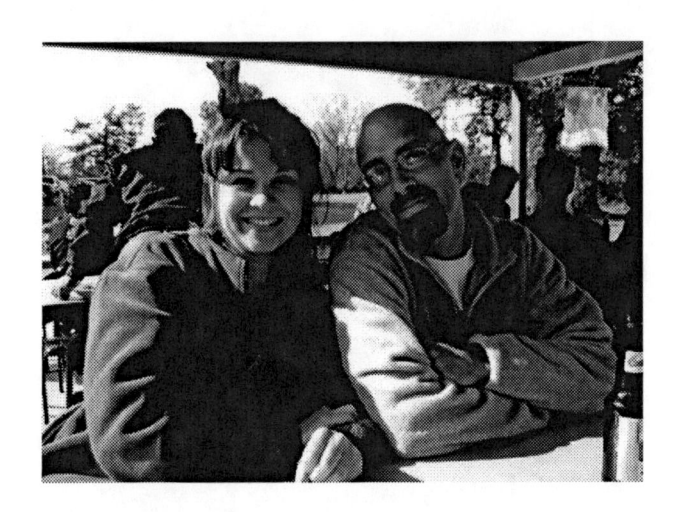

ABOUT THE AUTHOR:

Britton Ormiston is the proud mother of three beautiful children: Julia, 5 years; Nathaniel, 3 years and Justin, 6 months of age (on the cover). Britton and Marc have been married for one year and live in Athens, Georgia. Britton and Marc were middle school sweethearts and had the chance to rekindle a relationship after years of absence from one another. Marc has a beautiful 14 year old daughter, Hillary, from a previous marriage.

Britton is a graduate of Alexander High School, Douglasville, Georgia. She received her degree in Biology at UGA and currently works as a technician in the scientific field (molecular biology).

Britton's hopes and dreams span far beyond the scope of this book. She has a keen interest in assimilating common problems of motherhood in hopes of finding common sense solutions. Eventually, Britton would like to create a line of maternity clothing and help design better safety equipment for infants in the safety industry. She has a genuine love for mothers and an ability to try and seek out answers to help them come to happy terms with their new life in motherhood.

The First Guide to Help YOU Get Through Life After Pregnancy:

From the "Hospital Bed" to the "Rest of Your Life," this book is designed to help you understand and grow with the changes that occur in your life after your child is born.

Topics Include:

* Giving Birth and Hospital Care
* Being a parent for the first time
* At home with your new little one
* Daycare choices and decisions
* The Dreaded Back to Work
* Breastfeeding and Pumping at Work
* Best Buys, Good Tips and More
* When your child is sick
* Taking care of yourself first
* Can your marriage survive?
* This Is the Rest of Your Life

All the information you NEEDED to know, but no one ever told you! **Post Pregnancy, Tips for Survival, Marriage, and Day to Day Living** are just a few of the topics covered in this wonderful, well written book about how your **LIFE** really is **AFTER** your child's **BIRTH**.

Printed in the United States
68975LVS00005B/283-318